PRAISE FOR ANTHONY WILLIAM

"Celery juice is sweeping the globe. It's impressive how Anthony has created this movement and restored superior health in countless people around the world."

— Sylvester Stallone

"Anthony's understanding of foods, their vibrations, and how they interact with the body never ceases to amaze. Effortlessly he explains the potential harmony or disharmony in our choices in a way anyone can understand. He has a gift. Do your body a favor and treat yourself."

— Pharrell Williams, 12-time Grammy-winning artist and producer

"I've been drinking celery juice every morning for the last six months and feel great! I've noticed a huge difference in my energy levels and digestive system. I even travel now with my juicer so I don't miss out on my daily celery juice!"

— Miranda Kerr, international supermodel, founder and CEO of KORA Organics

"Anthony has turned numerous lives around for the better with the healing powers of celery juice."

— Novak Djokovic, #1-ranked tennis champion in the world

"All great gifts are bestowed with humility. Anthony is humble. And like all the right remedies, his are intuitive, natural, and balanced. These two make for a powerful and effective combination."

— John Donovan, CEO of AT&T Communications

"Anthony is a trusted source for our family. His work in the world is a light that has guided many to safety. He means so much to us."

— Robert De Niro and Grace Hightower De Niro

"While there is most definitely an element of otherworldly mystery to the work he does, much of what Anthony William shines a spotlight on—particularly around autoimmune disease—feels inherently right and true. What's better is that the protocols he recommends are natural, accessible, and easy to do."

— Gwyneth Paltrow, Oscar-winning actress, #1 *New York Times* best-selling author, founder and CEO of GOOP.com

"Anthony William is truly dedicated to sharing his knowledge and experience to spread the word of healing to all. His compassion and desire to reach as many people as he can to help them heal themselves is inspiring and empowering. Today, in a world of obsession with prescription medication, it is so refreshing to know that there are alternative options that truly work and can open a new door to health."

— Liv Tyler, star of *Harlots*, the *Lord of the Rings* trilogy, *Empire Records*

"I've been following Anthony for a while now and am always floored (but not surprised) at the success stories from people following his protocols . . . I have been on my own path of healing for many years, jumping from doctor to doctor and specialist to specialist. He's the real deal and I trust him and his vast knowledge of how the thyroid works and the true effects food has on our body. I have directed countless friends, family, and followers to Anthony because I truly believe he possesses knowledge that no doctor out there has. I am a believer and on a true path to healing now and am honored to know him and blessed to know his work.
Every endocrinologist needs to read his book on the thyroid!"

— Marcela Valladolid, chef, author, television host

"What if someone could simply touch you and tell you what it is that ails you? Welcome to the healing hands of Anthony William—a modern-day alchemist who very well may hold the key to longevity. His lifesaving advice blew into my world like a healing hurricane, and he has left a path of love and light in his wake. He is hands down the ninth wonder of the world."

— Lisa Gregorisch-Dempsey, *Extra* Senior Executive Producer

"Anthony William's God-given gift for healing is nothing short of miraculous."

— David James Elliott, *Impulse, Trumbo, Mad Men, CSI: NY*; star for ten years of *JAG*

"I am a doctor's daughter who has always relied on Western medicine to ameliorate even the smallest of woes. Anthony's insights opened my eyes to the healing benefits of food and how a more holistic approach to health can change your life."

— Jenny Mollen, actress and *New York Times* best-selling author of *I Like You Just the Way I Am*

"Anthony William is a gift to humanity. His incredible work has helped millions of people heal when conventional medicine had no answers for them. His genuine passion and commitment for helping people is unsurpassed, and I am grateful to have been able to share a small part of his powerful message in Heal."

— Kelly Noonan Gores, writer, director, and producer of the *Heal* documentary

"Anthony William is one of those rare individuals who uses his gifts to help people rise up to meet their full potential by becoming their own best health advocates . . . I witnessed Anthony's greatness in action firsthand when I attended one of his thrilling live events. I equate how spot-on his readings were with a singer hitting all the high notes. But beyond the high notes, Anthony's truly compassionate soul is what left the audience captivated. Anthony William is someone I am now proud to call a friend, and I can tell you that the person you hear on the podcasts and whose words fill the pages of best-selling books is the same person who reaches out to loved ones simply to lend support. This is not an act! Anthony William is the real deal, and the gravity of the information he shares through Spirit is priceless and empowering and much needed in this day and age!"

— Debbie Gibson, Broadway star, iconic singer-songwriter

"Anthony William has devoted his life to helping people with information that has truly made a substantial difference in the lives of many."

— Amanda de Cadenet, founder and CEO of The Conversation and the Girlgaze Project; author of *It's Messy* and *#girlgaze*

"I love Anthony William! My daughters Sophia and Laura gave me his book for my birthday, and I couldn't put it down. The Medical Medium has helped me connect all the dots on my quest to achieve optimal health. Through Anthony's work, I realized the residual Epstein-Barr left over from a childhood illness was sabotaging my health years later. Medical Medium has transformed my life."

— Catherine Bach, *The Young and the Restless*, *The Dukes of Hazzard*

"My recovery from a traumatic spinal crisis several years ago had been steady, but I was still experiencing muscle weakness, a tapped-out nervous system, as well as extra weight. A dear friend called me one evening and strongly recommended I read the book Medical Medium by Anthony William. So much of the information in the book resonated with me that I began incorporating some of the ideas, then I sought and was lucky enough to get a consultation. The reading was so spot-on, it has taken my healing to an unimagined, deeper, and richer level of health. My weight has dropped healthily, I can enjoy bike riding and yoga, I'm back in the gym, I have steady energy, and I sleep deeply. Every morning when following my protocols, I smile and say, 'Whoa, Anthony William! I thank you for your restorative gift . . . Yes!'"

— Robert Wisdom, *The Alienist*, *Flaked*, *Rosewood*, *Nashville*, *The Wire*, *Ray*

"In this world of confusion, with constant noise in the health and wellness field, I rely on Anthony's profound authenticity. His miraculous, true gift rises above it all to a place of clarity."

— Patti Stanger, host of *Million Dollar Matchmaker*

"I rely on Anthony William for my and my family's health. Even when doctors are stumped, Anthony always knows what the problem is and the pathway for healing."

— Chelsea Field, *NCIS: New Orleans*, *Secrets and Lies*, *Without a Trace*, *The Last Boy Scout*

"Anthony William brings a dimension to medicine that deeply expands our understanding of the body and of ourselves. His work is part of a new frontier in healing, delivered with compassion and with love."

— Marianne Williamson, #1 *New York Times* best-selling author of *Healing the Soul of America*, *The Age of Miracles*, and *A Return to Love*

"Anthony William is a generous and compassionate guide. He has devoted his life to supporting people on their healing path."

— Gabrielle Bernstein, #1 *New York Times* best-selling author of *The Universe Has Your Back*, *Judgment Detox*, and *Miracles Now*

"Information that WORKS. That's what I think of when I think of Anthony William and his profound contributions to the world. Nothing made this fact so clear to me as seeing him work with an old friend who had been struggling for years with illness, brain fog, and fatigue. She had been to countless doctors and healers and had gone through multiple protocols. Nothing worked. Until Anthony talked to her, that is . . . from there, the results were astounding. I highly recommend his books, lectures, and consultations. Don't miss this healing opportunity!"

— Nick Ortner, *New York Times* best-selling author of *The Tapping Solution for Manifesting Your Greatest Self* and *The Tapping Solution*

"Esoteric talent is only a complete gift when it's shared with moral integrity and love. Anthony William is a divine combination of healing, giftedness, and ethics. He's a real-deal healer who does his homework and shares it in true service to the world."

— Danielle LaPorte, best-selling author of *White Hot Truth* and *The Desire Map*

"Anthony is a seer and a wellness sage. His gift is remarkable. With his guidance I've been able to pinpoint and address a health issue that's been plaguing me for years."

— Kris Carr, *New York Times* best-selling author of *Crazy Sexy Juice*, *Crazy Sexy Kitchen*, and *Crazy Sexy Diet*

"Twelve hours after receiving a heaping dose of self-confidence masterfully administered by Anthony, the persistent ringing in my ears of the last year . . . began to falter. I am astounded, grateful, and happy for the insights offered on moving forward."

— Mike Dooley, *New York Times* best-selling author of *Infinite Possibilities* and scribe of *Notes from the Universe*

"Whenever Anthony William recommends a natural way of improving your health, it works. I've seen this with my daughter, and the improvement was impressive. His approach of using natural ingredients is a more effective way of healing."

— Martin D. Shafiroff, financial advisor, past recipient of #1 Broker in America ranking by WealthManagement.com and #1 Wealth Advisor ranking by Barron's

"Anthony William's invaluable advice on preventing and combating disease is years ahead of what's available anywhere else."

— Richard Sollazzo, M.D., New York board-certified oncologist, hematologist, nutritionist, and anti-aging expert and author of *Balance Your Health*

"Anthony William is the Edgar Cayce of our time, reading the body with outstanding precision and insight. Anthony identifies the underlying causes of diseases that often baffle the most astute conventional and alternative health-care practitioners. Anthony's practical and profound advice makes him one of the most powerfully effective healers of the 21st century."

— Ann Louise Gittleman, *New York Times* best-selling author of over 30 books on health and healing and creator of the highly popular Fat Flush detox and diet plan

"As a Hollywood businesswoman, I know value. Some of Anthony's clients spent over $1 million seeking help for their 'mystery illness' until they finally discovered him."

— Nanci Chambers, co-star of *JAG*; Hollywood producer and entrepreneur

"I had a health reading from Anthony, and he accurately told me things about my body only known to me. This kind, sweet, hilarious, self-effacing, and generous man—also so 'otherworldly' and so extraordinarily gifted, with an ability that defies how we see the world— has shocked even me, a medium! He is truly our modern-day Edgar Cayce, and we are immensely blessed that he is with us. Anthony William proves that we are more than we know."

— Colette Baron-Reid, best-selling author of *Uncharted* and TV host of *Messages from Spirit*

"Any quantum physicist will tell you there are things at play in the universe we can't yet understand. I truly believe Anthony has a handle on them. He has an amazing gift for intuitively tapping into the most effective methods for healing."

— Caroline Leavitt, *New York Times* best-selling author of *The Kids' Family Tree Book, Cruel Beautiful World, Is This Tomorrow,* and *Pictures of You*

MEDICAL MEDIUM

CELERY JUICE

THE MOST POWERFUL MEDICINE OF OUR TIME
HEALING MILLIONS WORLDWIDE

MEDICAL MEDIUM

CELERY JUICE

THE MOST POWERFUL MEDICINE OF OUR TIME
HEALING MILLIONS WORLDWIDE

ANTHONY WILLIAM

HAY HOUSE, INC.
Carlsbad, California • New York City
London • Sydney • New Delhi

Published in the United States by: Hay House, Inc.: www.hayhouse.com®
Published in Australia by: Hay House Australia Pty. Ltd.: www.hayhouse.com.au
Published in the United Kingdom by: Hay House UK, Ltd.: www.hayhouse.co.uk
Published in India by: Hay House Publishers India: www.hayhouse.co.in

Cover design: Vibodha Clark
Interior design: Bryn Starr Best
Indexer: Jay Kreider

Cataloging-in-Publication Data is on file at the Library of Congress

Hardcover ISBN: 978-1-4019-5765-0
e-book ISBN: 978-1-4019-5766-7

10 9 8 7 6 5 4 3 2 1
1st edition, May 2019

Printed in the United States of America

SUSTAINABLE FORESTRY INITIATIVE
Certified Chain of Custody
Promoting Sustainable Forestry
www.sfiprogram.org
SFI-01268

SFI label applies to the text stock

For the billions on the planet who have suffered
with any kind of health challenge, this one belongs to you.
It is your right to be heard, be taken seriously,
and have the freedom to heal.

— Anthony William, Medical Medium

"Celery juice is a beacon of light offered to us here on Earth, an answer for those who've given up on answers."

— Anthony William, Medical Medium

CONTENTS

"You are the greatest expert on your health, and your healing story counts. It counts for more than you know. Someone out there right now is waiting to hear your story so they can discover this life-changing medicine."

— Anthony William, Medical Medium

CHAPTER 1

Why Celery Juice?

Celery juice is helping millions of people heal.

Really? Celery juice? you may be thinking, if you haven't heard the buzz, or even if you have.

Really. Celery juice.

That unremarkable vegetable going limp in my refrigerator?

That's right. The overlooked, underestimated, underused herb (yes, herb) that you know from the occasional tuna salad, stuffing, or ants-on-a-log snack is far more powerful than anyone realizes—if you know how to apply it to your life.

For decades, I've been recommending celery juice as an unparalleled healing elixir. Whether someone is looking for relief from a specific health issue or for that secret tonic to help them get their energy and glow back, celery juice has been an answer to a prayer. For all that time, I've had the privilege of watching it turn people's lives around.

With the publication of my first health book, *Medical Medium*, I started sharing about celery juice with the wider world. I've

featured it in all three of my books since then, because it's so versatile that it's been relevant every single time. The Medical Medium community has amazed me by taking this healing information to heart. After discovering for themselves that celery juice actually works, community members from around the globe have been spreading the message and sharing their testimonials. By the tens of thousands, they've posted before-and-after photos—showing their clearer skin, brighter eyes, stronger bodies, renewed vitality—that would astound you. The stories behind them, some describing how celery juice actually saved their lives, are even more extraordinary. People who once were struggling and now are well have offered boundless encouragement to friends and strangers. We've started a movement.

With all this attention celery juice is getting, it may seem like a trend that's here today and will be gone tomorrow. Rest assured, this is no passing fad. It didn't take off because of funding, the way health trends do. It took off because people are actually healing. Celery juice is even more useful at this moment in time than it was when I started recommending it years ago. It will be even more essential decades into the future. Put this book aside, pick it back up years from now, and it will still contain the healing truth you need. It won't be outmoded by new theories on diet and nutrition; drinking celery juice will remain a critical action that you can incorporate into your life for health and vitality at any time. Other health trends come and go because they were never the answer to begin with. This is different: it's lasting and true.

ORIGINS OF CELERY JUICE

The first time that God led me to recommend celery juice was in 1975, to bring down the inflammation of a family member's back injury after she fell down a staircase. It was unheard of at the time. I also distinctly remember suggesting it in 1977 to help a friend of the family who had a severe case of acid reflux.

By the age of 13 and 14, I was working as a stock boy at the local supermarket. There, I would do health consultations for people who asked, and I would take them over to the produce aisle to pick out what they needed for their symptoms and illnesses. My boss asked what would help these people more. "Well," I said, "I need a juicer." So he purchased a juicer.

Whenever a customer's situation called for it—whether someone had arthritis, gout,

diabetes, gastrointestinal issues, or other symptoms and conditions—I would grab a head of celery from the produce section, wash it, run it through the juicer, and carry a big cup of straight celery juice to them. I was usually aiming for that magic number of 16 ounces, and I'd have them drink this herbal medicine right there in the aisle. If someone was sensitive, I'd have them take a few sips on the spot and then tell them to take a few more sips as they were shopping and finish it in the car or at home. My boss would charge only for the celery, directing checkers to ring up customers for one bunch of celery per juice. By the time customers left the store, some of them would already feel relief from their various ailments.

I heard one question over and over again: "Do you have anything to sweeten it up?" Many people hadn't even heard of juicing yet, so the concept of fresh vegetable juice, not to mention fresh celery juice, was entirely foreign. The ones who had heard of juicing wanted some carrot, apple, or beet for flavor. I would always say, "That would defeat the purpose. It would interfere with the healing mechanism, the sodium cluster salts." (You'll read more about these shortly.)

Sometimes parents would give the juice to their kids, too. If a child had a cough, I'd bring out some celery juice, and a mom would hand it to her child to sip. Parents trusted me because they saw it worked. Celery juice was such a powerful remedy that if a kid was screaming or crying after eating a bunch of candy in the store and I carried out some celery juice for the parent to offer the child, it would bring about sudden calm and happiness. It was an incredible stabilizer for blood sugar highs and lows.

I was constantly running back and forth to the juicer so I could clean it out and make more celery juice. Combined with the time I spent doing little health consultations for customers, that meant my boss had to shift responsibilities so that someone else could do the job I was supposed to be doing: stocking shelves. He was gracious about it. He said he'd never ordered so much celery for a produce department in his life.

As I got older, I started doing lectures in health food stores in different parts of the country. There I would stand, in rooms filled with anywhere from 50 to 500 people, teaching about the powerful healing benefits of straight celery juice. This was the 1990s. Very few people had juicers at home, so I would show them how to make celery juice in a blender by liquefying chopped celery and then straining it. When someone owned neither a juicer nor a blender, I would tell them to chew celery sticks and spit out the pulp. While it wasn't the same— no one can chew that much celery—it was something. I'd recommend that to avoid a tired jaw, they should chew portions of it throughout the day.

When I brought up celery juice, I'd often see people's jaws drop. It wasn't a popular juicing staple. The juices of the day were still made with beets, carrots, and apples, sometimes with cucumber thrown in there, and if you were lucky, a few stalks of celery. Plain celery juice made no sense to people. It didn't even seem palatable.

People at least connected to the idea of celery as healthy, because they had heard of chopping it up for salads and adding it to soups. Some people described a wholesome celery-and-carrot broth a grandmother used to make. Others had even heard of celery having an ancient medicinal history—although it should be noted that very often when we hear about historical use of celery across different cultures, we're actually hearing about celery *root*, also known as celeriac, which is a different plant altogether from the celery grown for its stalks. That's right; celery root and celery are two different plants in the same family. With celery root, which is often compared to a turnip in appearance, it's not a great idea to juice it, because the only way to get usable nutrients out of celery root is to cook it. In its raw state, celery root is not easily digestible. When cooked, celery root still won't give you what celery or celery juice can.

Even with people's different thoughts on celery—and let's face it, no one was thinking about celery all that much—the idea of celery *juice* was new when I started suggesting it. Celery and celery juice are two different concepts with two different meanings. Fresh celery juice had never been used on a medicinal level, and certainly not in these dosages. If someone juiced a head of celery alone, it was because they found one wilting in the fridge that they needed to use up before it went bad. Most likely, they added a few carrots or an apple to the juice.

So as I recommended celery juice, I was met with a fair amount of skepticism.

Mostly, I was met with the question "Celery . . . juice?" People were so convinced that celery was best as some sticks with dip or as one ingredient among many that it sometimes felt like a nearly impossible feat to convince anyone that plain and simple celery juice held the healing power that it did. Doctors and other practitioners would cast it off as a non-option.

Meanwhile, the results I was seeing in people who took it seriously were truly profound. I traveled around, continuing to show people how to make celery juice in mom-and-pop health food stores, large health food stores, small theaters, and even church basements, spreading the message of its healing powers for anything and everything that ailed them, along with other information that I share in the Medical Medium books.

After one demonstration in the early 1990s of how to blend and strain celery to make juice, during which I had also delivered what was practically a dissertation on its powers, a young woman in her late 20s approached me.

"I'm struggling with addiction," she told me. "Addiction to anything and everything. I have an addictive personality."

"Then I want you to drink thirty-two ounces of celery juice once a day," I told her.

A month later, I was back in that health food store giving another talk. Out of the crowd of 80 or 90 people, the young woman approached me again. "Do you remember me?" she asked.

"You were dealing with the addiction problem," I said. "How are you?"

"You cured me of my addictions," she answered.

"I did?"

"Yes," the woman replied. "You told me to drink celery juice."

"*Celery juice* healed you of your addictions," I said. "Don't stop drinking it."

"I've never gone through a month of my life without struggle before, not since I was a little girl," she said. "I'll never stop drinking it."

Through the years, I found that celery juice did have a special ability to break vicious cycles. Whether an addiction was to food such as cakes and cookies and chips, overeating in general, recreational drugs, prescription drugs, anger, smoking, or anything else, someone would often experience anxiety or depression first. And if someone wasn't anxious or depressed to begin with, an addiction could lead them to be. The pattern of thoughts and feelings that led to certain behaviors, and behaviors that led to certain thoughts and feelings, could feel unstoppable. Celery juice cut right in and offered relief from addiction, anxiety, and depression all at once, helping someone gain their footing again.

Still, there would always be the doubters. During those lectures, the looks on people's faces would often say, *Celery? How can this be possible? Celery is worthless.* Sometimes people would laugh. (They still do, although it's becoming harder and harder to find celery juice laughable as more and more individuals go public with their healing stories.) Some people sitting in my lectures or visiting my office didn't have any desire to stray from carrot juice or from relying on prescription drugs.

Others were open, saying, "I'm sick. I've been through hell. I could barely drag myself here today. I'm so bad off, I can barely stand in front of you." One thing was the same then as it is now: when someone is unwell, they'll pursue opportunities they never would have before.

"What have you tried?" I would ask.

"Everything. It didn't work. I'll try anything," they would say.

So I would suggest celery juice.

"Celery juice it is," these few brave souls would answer. "Even though it doesn't seem like it would work and I probably won't like the taste, I'll give it a shot."

The human desire to heal is so strong that people will break down any barrier, trying options outside of conventional and even alternative health belief systems in search of what will really make them better. For the people who really tried celery juice, the rewards were enormous. Those who followed the guidelines that you'll find in this book and then kept with it, making 16 ounces of celery juice on an empty stomach a part of their daily life, found themselves almost in shock at what it did for them. Finally, they started to recover their health and experience greater well-being than anyone knew was possible. It remained a secret health remedy that I kept recommending year after year. By the late 1990s, I'd seen celery juice help thousands of people. There wasn't a symptom, condition, illness, disorder, or disease that I didn't see benefit from celery juice. It never disappointed.

As the years passed, I kept on recommending celery juice. At the same time, the Medical Medium community was building. Home juicers and juice bars were becoming more popular, making celery juice more accessible. Between the time I started recommending celery juice as a child and when I started putting out books in 2015, I had offered health guidance to hundreds of thousands of people and seen celery juice act as a major foundational aspect for the healing of so many.

With the Medical Medium series came a new wave of community members. Celery juice had always been a truth I had been able to hand people, so I featured it in each and every book. It was that versatile and vital. Now that technology had advanced, as readers tried it and benefitted, they were able to post their stories and connect with and inspire each other. With an increasing number of people trying celery juice and sharing about it, the celery juice movement kept building momentum.

Suddenly, greater numbers of people were walking up to juice counters around the world asking for celery juice. People working behind those counters were baffled. "Plain celery juice?" Even though they were used to making all kinds of different juices for hours a day over many years, they'd never heard anything like it and couldn't understand why anyone would want it. Grocery stores started selling out of celery as folks who liked to juice it at home stocked up. Produce managers were similarly shocked at the sudden celery demand.

Celery juice kept working for people, so the demand continued.

Now celery juice has finally made its way into the mainstream, solely because it works. It appears on juice menus and has starred in article after article. As heartening as it is that more and more people are benefiting, with all this attention on celery juice has come some misinformation. It's gotten a little more confusing for those who are looking for guidance to determine what they should believe about celery juice and which advice they should follow. With this book, my aim is to provide a clear guide to celery juice from the original source, one that answers as many questions as possible and covers celery juice's healing benefits like never before, so you can move forward with certainty and clarity.

RECONSIDER CELERY

Before we get into the amazing benefits of celery juice—as well as critical guidance about how to make it work best for you—we need to talk about celery for a moment. It doesn't have the most thrilling reputation. We think of it as useful, sure. A nice vehicle for peanut butter and raisins, a crunchy addition to egg salad, a good ingredient in soup stock, a garnish for buffalo wings or a Bloody Mary cocktail. We've heard of models eating celery to control weight. We consider it vaguely healthy, mainly because it's low in calories, or even nourishing, if we were the lucky recipients of a grandparent's vegetable broth. If suddenly you became

part of a special task force to locate the next great medicine on earth, though, you would probably go looking in the jungle. Celery wouldn't even enter your consciousness, even though it's one of the planet's great answers.

I understand if it's a little difficult to believe that celery juice could be quite as beneficial as it is. That ordinary green bundle that we've walked past a million times at the grocery store? The one we always forget to use up, because we only need a stick or two at a time? How could *that* be an undiscovered superfood? Really, it's an undiscovered *miracle* food. If you choose to keep viewing celery as an unassuming sidekick ingredient—if you're not truly seeing celery for what it is and what it can do—celery juice will still help you and work for you. Trouble is, you could give up on it too soon. And how is it going to aid you if you don't give it an honest try? If you want to push celery aside as too humble, know that you're pushing aside your own healing process. If you think of it only as the annoying little bits in your tuna salad, you're missing a critical opportunity.

If we want to connect with why it's worth trying celery juice more than once or twice, then we need to see celery in a new light. We need to know that it holds real potency and has the ability to help us reach new levels of health. Looking at celery with disrespect translates to disrespecting your healing process, and that's not fair to you. We're taught to have respect for ourselves and others—it's part of life in this world. The ultimate respect we can show is to this miraculous, powerhouse herb, because doing so is saying, "I want to heal." It's saying, "I want my loved ones to get better."

It can be easy for someone who thinks they're healthy to be skeptical or wary of celery juice. If that's you, and you feel you don't need celery juice in your life, please at least respect the stories from those who have healed from it. Consider the people who have suffered and seen celery juice quite seriously save their lives. Try not to fall into the mind-set that it's just juice. Try to think of the chronically ill and their return to health thanks to celery juice, or people's experiences of saving the health of their children, other family, and friends. Try to think of those who have used celery juice as one of their main tools to reverse the worst skin conditions, terrifying migraines, or the horrendous fatigue that was holding them back from living. Please keep an open heart toward those who are using celery juice to heal.

Nobody has assurance that they're never going to become ill or develop a symptom someday. We come into this world with toxins and pathogens already in our bodies, and we're exposed to new toxins and pathogens on a daily basis. Even with positive thinking and efforts to be our best self and attract goodness, we can't always control the various obstacles in our path through life. Sometimes we step in a pothole, we trip, and we fall. When that happens, celery juice is one of our greatest allies for recovery. Remember that it's sitting there waiting for you in the future,

should something ever happen with your health. Or—use celery juice to ensure you don't let something happen. Not being actively sick doesn't automatically mean that you're well. You may not want to wait until you've reached a critical state of illness years from now, a state that has finally led you to see celery juice's value. By that point, you'll have so much more progress to make. Celery juice is here for you right now as a preventative, an important way of preserving your physical and mental state and protecting who you are. Turning to it today and keeping up with it on a daily basis will add precious time to your life, and every extra moment counts. Celery juice is one of the greatest tools for becoming your strongest, most wonderful self. Give celery juice a chance, and it will work for you like nothing and no one else ever has.

That majestic plant that can take your healing further along than ever before won't be found deep in the Amazon. It's already in front of you. Celery is a miracle that's been sitting patiently on the grocery store shelf, waiting for its day in the sun, waiting to do what it was always supposed to do. All it needed was to be seen, juiced on its own, and consumed on an empty stomach. (And always remember that: when we're talking about celery juice, we are talking about pure, straight, unadulterated celery juice consumed on an empty stomach. By the end of this book, you'll be an expert on why.) Now, finally, celery juice can be recognized for the power it truly holds to help you move forward with your life and prosper.

HOW THIS BOOK WORKS

This book is designed to ignite the global celery juice movement while dying out the fire of chronic symptoms and illness. It's here to provide a viable, powerful, foundational tool for the billions of people on the planet suffering from long-term health issues. That's right: billions. And we're not just talking about half of the people on earth suffering, either. Almost three-quarters of Earth's population struggles with at least one persistent symptom or condition, and the remaining one-quarter will develop symptoms and illnesses if we stay on this trajectory. Without intervention, soon everybody on the planet is going to be suffering from a chronic health problem. Celery juice is meant to be that intervention, that first, accessible step people can take toward righting their health. This book is here to offer you answers to all your celery juice questions so that you can use it to reverse your own chronic illness, to protect friends and family from developing illness, or to offer loved ones the opportunity to reverse illness.

To start with, in the next chapter, we'll cover the benefits of celery juice. Here you'll find out just why celery juice holds the value it does. You'll read about pathogen-fighting sodium cluster salts, gut-soothing digestive enzymes, endocrine-balancing plant hormones, immune-boosting vitamin C, and more. Discovering what celery juice has to offer will give you even more incentive to stick with it. Understanding what the body needs and how it heals will activate the healing process that much more.

If you're struggling with a symptom, illness, or other health complaint, you'll take particular interest in Chapter 3, "Relief from Your Symptoms and Conditions." Find out about the true causes of dozens of health issues at the same time you discover how celery juice specifically helps each one. As I always say, solving the mystery of what's been holding you back can be a key part of moving past it.

Chapter 4, "How to Make Celery Juice Work for You," is where you'll find instructions for how to make celery juice, how much to drink (with children's guidelines, too), and when to drink it. For example, having a shot of celery juice here and there, while it will help in some way, is not likely to have a noticeable effect on your health. Most people's bodies are so overloaded that sporadic small dosages won't cut it. We need precise guidance on timing and amounts, and that's what this chapter offers. And that's just the beginning. There are so many other tips and answers packed in Chapter 4, including how to fit celery juice into your exercise or supplement routine, advice on picking out a juicer, whether it's okay to drink celery juice when pregnant or breastfeeding, why you actually need to separate celery from its fiber to unlock its potency, and what it is about drinking celery juice on an empty stomach that's so important. This chapter is a vital resource that I expect you'll want to refer back to from time to time.

Next we get to the Celery Juice Cleanse in Chapter 5. If you're looking for a simple structure that will help you stay on track with celery juice, the handful of daily steps outlined in this chapter will prime celery juice to work even better for you. This cleanse builds on the Liver Rescue Morning from my previous book, *Liver Rescue,* so if you've already tried that, you'll find these steps very natural.

Chapter 6, "Healing and Detox Answers," addresses some of the questions that come up around how long celery juice takes to make a difference as well as how it affects the body while it's working. There are a lot of misconceptions in this area, and it's important to know how to interpret your body's responses to celery juice. Especially because when some people first try celery juice, they may experience a healing reaction as the juice kills off bugs and scrubs the system clean. This can entail, for example, a funny taste in the mouth, additional body odor, or feeling the need to urinate more frequently. When this happens, they're still moving forward. So are the people who don't experience these types of healing reactions. This chapter is here to help you understand your own healing process and offer support throughout it.

In Chapter 7, "Rumors, Concerns, and Myths," we'll cover just what the title suggests. The celery juice movement has a purity and integrity to it—celery juice's popularity took off solely because people found that it helped them, and these gracious souls decided to spread the word. It took off because it got results. That means that those affiliated with funding-backed trends can find celery juice threatening, while those who approach life with skepticism distrust the buzz. As a result, certain doubts and misinformation about celery juice have arisen. This chapter is here to address them directly. Whether you're looking to set your own mind at ease or be ready for others' questions about celery juice, turn here for answers.

Whatever diet trends you follow—whether low-carb, high-fat, high-protein, vegan, plant-based, keto, or paleo—or healing modalities you believe in—whether Ayurvedic medicine, traditional Chinese medicine, conventional medicine, alternative medicine, or functional medicine—celery juice works with them and should be a part of your life. If you keep using it long term, it can provide even more results. Then, if you want to take your healing to the next level, you'll find more ideas in Chapter 8, "More Healing Guidance." Celery juice is an incredible beacon of light that can help provide someone with their initial rounds of recovery; with all the fads and trends out there, no other health remedy can give you results at the very root of the problem as powerfully or rapidly as celery juice. All on its own, it can deliver someone results for the first time in 10, 15, or 20 years of being sick. At the same time, celery juice is only one foundational tool to stabilize you and put you on the healing path. There's a lot more real, effective health guidance where celery juice came from. As celery juice has gained more and more attention, more confusion has arisen around it. The other health guidance you need in order to get better—the true guidance, not the theories or trends—has often gotten lost as certain platforms try to claim celery juice as their own. That's a disservice to the mom, dad, child, college student, professional, or grandparent struggling with a new diagnosis who needs to know what else will actually get them better. If you want your progress to take you all the way through recovery, you need more information to support your healing alongside celery juice: information from the same source where celery juice originated. Chapter 8 is here to guide you. It's imperative to know that the celery juice movement stems from this source, so that you know this is where you'll find the other healing information that supports it and works with it.

I get that celery and celery juice aren't always available. Sometimes storms wipe out a crop or you're traveling without a juicer, with no source of fresh celery juice in sight. Chapter 9 moves on to alternatives to celery juice for those times when you're in a pinch. This chapter hands you a few different options to get you through until you can access celery juice again.

Finally, if you're wondering where the evidence is to back up celery juice as such a valuable healing remedy, you'll find an explanation of where I get my information in Chapter 10, "A Healing Movement." You can also look to the millions of people around the world who are drinking celery juice and getting better. Ask them their stories, read the ones already out there, or try it yourself. You will find compelling proof of celery juice's potency.

YOUR WINNING APPROACH

Celery juice is for wherever we are in life. People ebb and flow with their food choices, changing diets constantly as they bounce across different trendy, name-brand food protocols and regimens or settle into familiar routines that don't follow any rules. Wherever you are with food, you can incorporate celery juice. It's always a winning approach because it's a real answer to getting better that's not attached to any belief system.

What I see in people who have brought celery juice into their lives, more even than the physical improvements, is the stronger light coming from within. Remember, celery juice itself is a beacon of light offered to us here on Earth, an answer for those who've given up on answers. If you're new to celery juice, welcome. If you're one of the people who has shone your light and spread the word about celery juice, I thank you. Each reader, whether a celery juice newbie or already its greatest champion, is a vital member of this healing movement.

When I wrote in *Life-Changing Foods* that "I could go on and on about the benefits of celery juice for all manner of ills. It is one of the greatest healing tonics of all time," I meant it. Here we are. With this book, packed with brand-new information on celery juice and answers to dozens of your questions, I hope to honor every one of you.

CHAPTER 2

Celery Juice Benefits

Celery is uncharted territory. It's understudied. There is not yet enough research about what consuming celery regularly can do for us to reveal all of its benefits, so nobody realizes what a nutritional powerhouse it is.

That's just celery itself. You can imagine, then, that if regular celery is understudied, celery *juice*—not long ago considered obscure—has certainly not gotten its due scientifically. Research tends to lump celery and celery juice together, considering them the same. If the rare study is actually done on celery, the reasoning goes that it should be good enough to indicate the nutritional components of fresh celery juice. That's far from true. Celery juice is an herbal extract on a level above plain celery. It deserves to be studied separately so that its unique healing properties can be witnessed and documented.

As of this writing, the world is still waiting for a rigorous, peer-reviewed study on the effects of drinking 16 ounces of fresh celery juice daily on an empty stomach.

When researchers finally do take this on, the design of the study will be critical. Attempts to make it double-blind could lead technicians to mask the flavor or color of the celery juice so participants won't know what they're drinking and researchers won't know what they're handing out—and those additives will compromise celery juice's purity and therefore potency. Or they could try to get around the issue by administering some sort of celery extract pill. Again, that's not going to offer what 16 ounces of fresh celery juice does. If study results come out that cast doubt on celery juice's efficacy, pay close attention to the methodology. Only the most respectful, stringent standards will do.

Any celery research we do hear about is focused on celery sticks, celery leaf, celery seeds, or celery powder reconstituted into a liquid. None of these do for us what freshly juiced celery does. Further, the studies aren't focused on reversing disease in humans. Some of them apply to preserving meat and are then taken out of context to get people worried about nitrates and nitrites. (Set your mind at ease in Chapter 7, "Rumors, Concerns, and Myths.") Those studies that are health-related mostly use rodents. And remember, a stalk of celery being examined in a lab does not mean that celery juice is being studied. Again, they're not one and the same; they're worlds apart. While that may be hard to swallow (so to speak), they really are different. Chewing on some stalks of celery neither gives us the quantity of nutrients nor unlocks the potency that juicing it does.

Medical research and science will someday catch up with the millions of people who have found healing with celery juice—the ones who have discovered more energy and stamina than ever, reversed chronic and acute conditions alike, and gotten their lives back. They will someday discover that celery juice is not a fad or a hiccup. They will find that it is—objectively—a healing medicine of our time.

Until they reach that discovery, they're likely to raise fear around the idea of something wrong with celery juice. Our world works a little backward sometimes. We always have to remember that as honorable as the pursuit of science is, it doesn't exist on a plane above humans. Science is a human pursuit, not the fully independent, impartial process we sometimes idealize it to be. Scientists are under enormous pressure. To run studies, labs need money, and that doesn't always come from the most honest or impartial sources. Funding and vested interests can affect outcomes or interpretations of results. (More on this in Chapter 10, "A Healing Movement.")

Because fresh celery juice is so simple, not terribly scalable or profitable, and threatens the status quo of moneymaking health products, it's most likely that an interest group will fund a study that purports to find a problem with celery juice in order to try to get this movement to fade away. The industries don't like rogue disease-reversing methods that work—*rogue* meaning untamed by patents and unchained from the monetary system. Celery juice can't be turned into pills and then bottled and withheld from people unless they pay large sums of money. Not that this will stop anyone. There is still the bandwagon of those trying to capitalize on celery and celery juice without a true understanding of what it's really doing for the chronically ill—people who deserve to finally find this answer that can bring them hope and healing.

Eventually, people will come back to the truth. They will find that even with all this noise, celery juice—real, pure, fresh celery juice, not attempts to preserve or alter it—keeps working. They will find that any fear was unfounded and that celery juice is and always will be a miracle remedy.

And they will find that there are specific reasons why celery juice helps you heal: major components of celery juice that are responsible for this global healing movement. You'll notice many dietitians and nutritionists saying that the reason people benefit from celery is that it's rich in vitamins A and K. Yes, it does contain vitamins such as A and K. So does virtually every vegetable and herb. People aren't having miracle recoveries because of those other foods, though. These nutrition stats alone don't offer insights into just why this herbal remedy is turning people's lives around, and that's why skeptics remain so confused. There are aspects of celery juice's power that nobody knows about yet. Those undiscovered benefits are what we're here to explore.

SODIUM CLUSTER SALTS

You're going to see talk of sodium in this book, most often of *sodium cluster salts*. If you have a shaky history with sodium and the word makes you nervous, let me assure you that the sodium in celery juice is beneficial. Even if you're on a low-sodium diet, you can still have celery juice. It's not like eating a food that's had table salt—or even healthier salts like Himalayan rock salt or Celtic sea salt—thrown on it. While your body does not see regular salt added to food as a friend, it accepts the sodium from celery juice as one of its own.

Celery juice is on your side. It actually removes crystallized toxic salts that have been in your organs for years. Now, if you get a blood test when you're on celery juice, it could show elevated sodium. What the test is really detecting are these old, toxic salts that celery juice is rounding up and sending out of your body. Plus, chances are you haven't given up table salt, so the blood analysis is picking up on that salt in your

system as well. Blood testing isn't nuanced enough to pick up on the difference.

A blood test could detect some sodium from celery juice, too, although it's going to be what I call *macro sodium*, a common form of plant sodium that's entirely healthy and needed. It's so beneficial and balancing that it doesn't spike the blood—meaning that if a blood test is displaying elevated sodium, celery juice's sodium isn't causing it. Elevated sodium levels are also not caused by celery juice's sodium cluster salts. A blood test isn't sensitive enough to pick up on celery juice's sodium cluster salts; testing isn't geared to find them, because they're a subgroup of sodium that hasn't been discovered yet by research and science.

So celery juice's beneficial macro sodium only stabilizes the blood; it won't lead to high sodium readings. Again, though, it could take a little time to get to those stabilized readings, or they could come and go, because (1) it's really easy to overindulge in table salt, since it's practically everywhere, and that's going to show up on a blood test, and (2) periodically, celery juice is going to be clearing out pockets of old, toxic salt as it reaches them deep in the organs, and that's going to throw off blood test interpretations.

Celery juice's complicated structures of beneficial sodium are elevated above other types, with different jobs and responsibilities. This is an entirely different make and model of sodium. It serves as a critical component of neurotransmitters—better said, it's the ultimate neurotransmitter chemical. It's what makes celery juice the most powerful electrolyte beverage on the planet. Nothing can surpass or even equal it.

Let's talk more about the undiscovered subgroup of celery juice's sodium that I call *sodium cluster salts*. "Sodium" and "salt" may sound a bit redundant, and yet it communicates that they are mineral salts that cluster around the macro sodium in celery juice. That is, sodium cluster salts are a separate acting group of compounds that surround the element we know as sodium in celery, all of it arranged in a structured form, almost like our solar system. Trace minerals also reside in these living, moving clusters. Some trace minerals are bonded to the sodium cluster salts themselves, and some simply float inside the clusters.

There is information for us within these clusters. That's rare. For the most part, plants are all about themselves. (Sound a bit like humans sometimes?) The information they contain is largely geared to sustaining themselves in their habitat, to accessing nourishment, to survival. Celery is different. Some of its information is for us, or for other animals consuming it. Sodium cluster salts aren't there as a defense mechanism or to keep the celery healthy as it's growing; they aren't there to keep the plant alive. They're for us. Sodium cluster salts contain information for our own well-being that's activated when it enters our bodies. Information from the plant—the herb—itself and information from the sun as the plant was growing. Information about its purpose and how it can help the creature consuming it. Information about the complex job of extending

our lives. Even if celery is grown in poor soil, it will still possess its cluster salts.

All salt is not the same. Although it can be easy to believe that sodium is sodium whether it's in the ocean, a vegetable, soil, rock, or a salt lake, it's not. If viewing it properly in a chemist's lab, a technician would discover the various salts contained within the sodium in celery juice. That technician would find that the salts cluster around each other, acting as one—as the sodium in no other herb, vegetable, or mineral does. Not even the salt in the ocean behaves in the particular way that this humble herb's does.

The sodium cluster salts in celery juice are able to neutralize toxins as they're floating through the bloodstream and organs. That means that when the cluster salts touch them, they disarm the troublemakers, making them more friendly and acceptable to the body and less toxic, so that they don't do harm to our human cells and organ tissue.

Toxic heavy metals are a particular type of toxin that celery juice's sodium cluster salts take on. Heavy metals have a destructive, active charge to them that causes the metals to be damaging to liver cells, brain cells, and other cells throughout the body. Cluster salts defuse the charge, rendering them inactive and less aggressive, specifically disarming toxic heavy metals such as copper, mercury, and aluminum.

Sodium cluster salts also fight off unwanted bacteria and viruses. (You'll read so much more about this ability throughout the next chapter.) Tricky bugs such as strep can't become resistant or immune to them, the way they can to pharmaceutical antibiotics, so the cluster salts keep on working as you drink celery juice over time. Celery juice's mineral salts are able to kill off bacterial, fungal, and viral overgrowth as they travel through the small intestine and colon, and even once they're absorbed into the bloodstream and pulled up into the liver through the hepatic portal vein. They're an incredible antiseptic in this way, enhancing your entire body's immune system.

These mineral salts are also able to support the liver in producing bile. That's partly because the cluster salts enter the bile to make it stronger and partly because the celery juice rejuvenates the liver overall, allowing it to function properly and produce bile more efficiently. This is one aspect of what makes celery juice extraordinary for the liver.

To recap: The sodium in celery juice is suspended in living water within the celery. Inside that living water are sodium cluster salts, tightly connected to it. So the cluster salts surround and suspend sodium, and they're also varieties of sodium themselves. The different forms of sodium become one and they're also separate. That's how celery juice is structured. Medical research and science haven't identified this yet because they haven't tried to look beyond "celery has salt." It's not nearly that simple. If they analyze it superficially, it's going to look like salt. If they analyzed it further, they would be able to separate out and identify the different varieties of sodium within celery juice. And then they would be closer to identifying all that these sodium cluster salts do for our health.

Rather than having to wait decades for these medical answers, you already hold them in your hands. You'll find out so much about the surprising and potent benefits of sodium cluster salts throughout this book, particularly in the next chapter, "Relief from Your Symptoms and Conditions."

COFACTOR MICRO TRACE MINERALS

A moment ago, I mentioned the trace minerals that are part of the sodium cluster salt clusters. To get more specific, I call them *cofactor micro trace minerals*. These undiscovered trace minerals, some of which are bonded to the cluster salts and some of which are free-floating within the living chemical compounds, are highly beneficial for digestion. This is in part because they help restore a dimension of hydrochloric acid that medical research and science haven't yet realized is lacking. That's right— our stomach's hydrochloric acid is actually a complex seven-acid blend, and celery juice helps bring acids back when they've diminished. Here's how: Cofactor micro trace minerals rejuvenate stomach gland tissue by entering and feeding the cells of the glands, providing them with newfound energy so they can function optimally. (Our stomach gland cells are only as good as the minerals of which they're made up.) In turn, stomach glands are able to produce the full seven-acid blend in its most potent form, which allows the gastric acid to kill off unproductive bugs in the stomach, duodenum, and farther down the small intestinal tract. This is not to be confused with the pathogen-killing ability of sodium cluster salts themselves, which travel down the intestinal tract directly, disarming viruses and bacteria as they go. Cofactor trace minerals are helping your stomach create better hydrochloric acid to defend itself. That's what gives your gastric juices more potency to kill off unproductive bugs in the gut.

Different parts of your body have their own individual immune systems, too, and celery juice's cofactor trace minerals help them out as well. For example, these trace minerals strengthen your liver's personalized immune system, lending strength to its lymphocytes (white blood cells) to fight off invaders like strep. Your liver also uses celery juice's trace minerals to create a chemical weapon that outright harms unproductive bugs like strep—playing offense, not just defense.

ELECTROLYTES

What makes electrolytes so important? Your body runs on electricity. An electrolyte allows electricity to flow, and it passes information from cell to cell throughout your entire body. Electrolytes help cells receive oxygen. They provide cells with the ability to detoxify and eliminate poisons. They're part of the cell-to-cell communication of every function in your body: they help you

think, *I need to go to the bathroom*, for example, and then help get you there.

When we hear that drinks contain electrolytes, that doesn't automatically mean they're in completed, active, and alive form. Many times, they're partial electrolytes, separated trace minerals, or minerals. They're building blocks. Celery juice contains complete living electrolytes: sodium cluster salts in full completion. This is what makes celery juice the ultimate electrolyte source.

Neurotransmitter chemicals in our brain are made up of electrolytes. It takes the complete electrolytes in celery juice entering the body to fully restore neurotransmitter chemicals so they can bring life back to neurotransmitters that have become dehydrated, dysfunctional, and practically nonexistent. (A neurotransmitter is like an empty beehive. Neurotransmitter chemicals are like the bees that bring life to the hive.) Other sources restore neurotransmitter chemicals only by chance—scraps of partial electrolytes float by, and they incrementally collect. A little bit of potassium from this food, a little bit of magnesium from this drink, a little bit of sodium from this sea salt. These building blocks end up scattered in our bodies, and while the body is always trying to make use of them, we're usually deficient, and it's the complete electrolytes in celery juice that really bring life to our blood supply and organs as they float along. No other food, herb, or beverage can supply every activated electrolyte needed at once to form a complete neurotransmitter chemical; only celery juice can. And the complete electrolytes in celery juice provide neurotransmitters with the ultimate revitalization inside the brain. Once a celery juice electrolyte lands on a neuron and gets wired in, an electrical impulse will ignite it, and it's like a light switch has been turned on. This in turn offers us unparalleled relief. More than complete electrolytes, they're complete neurotransmitter chemicals, performing a takeover and restoration so our neurotransmitters can be put back in working order and we can function at our best. And because celery juice's electrolytes contain everything at once, the body doesn't have to work at gathering minerals in hopes of sustaining itself. It's handed the complete package, ready to go.

PLANT HORMONES

Celery juice contains a specific undiscovered plant hormone that feeds and replenishes every single gland in the endocrine system, among them the pancreas, hypothalamus, pituitary gland, pineal gland, thyroid, and adrenals. It's one of the reasons why celery juice is such a miracle at providing balance in the body; it's a big part of why people heal and recover with celery juice.

It's also one of the reasons why celery juice is like a magic healing button for those with autoimmune disorders: because everyone sick with an autoimmune or other viral issue is up against endocrine challenges. Celery juice's sodium cluster salts and this plant hormone together are like a one-two punch for autoimmune disease. From one side, you've got the cluster salts knocking back the pathogenic activity responsible for autoimmune conditions. Then you've got the celery juice plant hormone helping out the endocrine glands such as the thyroid by entering, strengthening, and stabilizing them. If a gland is slightly hypo (underactive), this hormone infusing it over time—because someone is drinking celery juice every day—gives the gland enough dosages to start coming back to balance. If a gland is hyper (overactive), those regular infusions will help calm it down. This plant hormone is also very useful for the endocrine inconsistencies, from mild to severe, that everyone experiences, not just those sick with autoimmune issues. From weakened adrenals to an underactive thyroid, endocrine struggles are rampant, and this celery juice plant hormone addresses them.

Really, celery juice contains an abundance of plant hormones not yet studied or categorized by medical research and science. Only one specific plant hormone provides these endocrine benefits, although a few others do offer benefits to the human body. Another beneficial plant hormone in celery juice is one that strengthens the reproductive system in humans—both men and women. This plant hormone helps regulate and balance the production of reproductive hormones and also stimulate the reproductive system in general. This is unlike other plants in the plant kingdom, where the hormones they contain are solely for the plant and its growing process. While some of celery's hormones are for the plant itself, it also contains plant hormones that are actually medicine for us. This is an aspect of the herb that raises celery above all the other herbs and vegetables to stabilize the systems of those who are ill or suffering. Celery is that unique. It offers the ultimate plant medicine.

Many herbal remedies cannot be consumed in high quantities. That's another reason why celery juice is such a gift, changing lives: we can safely drink larger amounts of it, which means receiving higher dosages of the medicine it provides. (More on how much celery juice is appropriate in the next chapter.) It's going to take decades before science funds the research to discover the medicinal plant hormones in celery—and then to study the good they're capable of in the human body. Until then, you know, and you can put them to use right now.

DIGESTIVE ENZYMES

The digestive enzymes in celery juice aren't ones that focus on breaking down food in the stomach. Their function is much more surprising and unique. Instead, they're like little capsules that are activated by pH change when they enter the small intestinal tract. No other food has enzymes that work quite like this.

You don't need a ton of enzymes from celery juice to make a huge digestive impact, because they have a (positive) infectious quality. A celery juice enzyme is like a comedian onstage at a comedy club telling a joke that starts a whole crowd laughing. That is, one celery juice enzyme can reignite, revive, and reactivate multiple weakened digestive enzymes from other sources that are hanging around in the small intestine.

Some of these other enzymes come from food. Many of them come from the pancreas, and many unknown enzymes come from the liver. Producing this third type of digestive enzyme is an undiscovered chemical function of the liver; not to be confused with the "liver enzymes" you hear about in blood tests, these digestive enzymes are produced by the liver and then released into the small intestinal tract through bile. These are completely different from pancreatic enzymes; to discover the liver's digestive enzymes, you'd have to know what you're looking for, and probing this is not a priority for medical research and science right now. In the decades to come, though, research and science will discover that these digestive enzymes exist within the bile coming from our livers.

When the liver is overburdened and weakened—and most everyone's is—its digestive enzymes are not as strong as they're meant to be, so they can't assist with functions such as digestion and the dispersal of fats to their intended degree. Celery juice enzymes re-stimulate these weary enzymes so they can do their job. Plus, celery juice enzymes re-stimulate enzymes from food that have found their habitat in the small intestine; plus, celery juice itself is a reviver of the liver, meaning that drinking it leads the liver to produce stronger bile-related digestive enzymes in the first place; plus, celery juice enzymes help strengthen the pancreas and ignite pancreatic enzymes; *plus*, the enzymes in celery juice themselves are profoundly powerful for the breakdown, digestion, and assimilation of certain nutrients that neither bile nor hydrochloric acid addresses, because the digestion process is that complex. Adds up to quite a lot, doesn't it? There's more.

Remember, medical research and science still don't know everything that happens to food when it enters the stomach. They have theories. They don't yet have all the answers. When we're talking about the digestive enzymes in celery juice that perform these functions, we're not talking about only one type of enzyme. We're talking about three varieties. Science hasn't discovered them yet, so they don't have names. I could call them Spring, Summer, and Fall for fun. Once they're found, researchers could just as easily end up naming them 374, 921, and 813.

Regardless, these three undiscovered enzymes exist in celery juice. As you just read about, they are life preservers to tired, weakened, diminished digestive enzymes from other sources. They're also partially responsible for the reduction of unproductive acid and mucus inside the intestinal tract. Most people's upper small intestines are filled with this mucus and toxic acid, and these enzymes are critical for diffusing, reducing, and balancing the acid while eating away, breaking down, and dissolving the mucus, essentially pushing it out of the intestinal tract. Once the mucus is gone, celery juice's sodium cluster salts have much easier access to microbes, so they can destroy these bugs such as strep (responsible for SIBO—small intestinal bacterial overgrowth), other unproductive bacteria, and viruses in the small intestine. (I know some sources often believe that parasites are in the gut, too. If you truly had a parasite, you would know—you would be so sick that you'd find yourself in the hospital. That said, if you still believe that a parasite is behind your gut trouble, then yes, celery juice enzymes would address that, too.)

Celery juice actually contains well over two dozen varieties of enzymes, most of them undiscovered and involved in the breakdown of waste matter inside the intestinal tract. It's the three special enzymes—Spring, Summer, and Fall, if you'd like—that specifically take action in the small intestinal tract, performing many of the behind-the-scenes functions of celery juice that people don't realize are responsible for making them feel better to such an extent. Depending on where celery is grown and what variety it is and whether it was watered more and given more nutritious dirt, a planting could have a higher volume of these three digestive enzymes, meaning that you could end up with even more potent benefits from a given batch. A planting of celery could also have extra amounts of only one or two of those specific enzymes. It varies. All celery, no matter what, will still have the three special enzymes.

ANTIOXIDANTS

One of the functions of the antioxidants in celery juice is to remove fatty deposits from around toxic heavy metal deposits in your body. Common places for heavy metal deposits are the brain and the liver. Fatty deposits cling to toxic heavy metal deposits like suction cups, and when fatty deposits and toxic heavy metals touch like this, it causes the metals to oxidize. Toxic heavy metals possess a destructive charge, which is part of what causes them to react to fatty deposits and other toxic heavy metals so aggressively and create oxidation in the process. Essentially, we're talking about metals rusting in the body, leading to corrosive runoff that's damaging to nearby tissue. Fatty deposits, which are highly absorbent, also draw in this toxic discharge, which is extremely fat soluble. As a result, the fatty deposit becomes highly toxic and can then act as fuel for the Epstein-Barr virus (EBV), shingles, human herpesvirus 6 (HHV-6), or any other kind of pathogen that may reach the brain and cause a myriad of symptoms and conditions, some of them diagnosed as autoimmune disease.

Heavy metals and heavy metal oxidation are undiscovered leading causes of brain fog, memory loss, depression, anxiety, bipolar disorder, attention-deficit/hyperactivity disorder (ADHD), and autism, as well as severe mental and physical deterioration such as Alzheimer's, ALS (amyotrophic lateral sclerosis), and Parkinson's. Celery juice's antioxidants help prevent metals from decaying by removing fatty deposits from around heavy metal deposits and also specially coating the heavy metals to discourage oxidation. Sodium cluster salts attached to celery juice's antioxidants defuse toxic heavy metals' destructive charge, rendering the heavy metals much less aggressive. With the destructive charge neutralized, celery juice's special antioxidants can stop oxidation much more effectively. It's yet one more of celery juice's unique, unknown abilities to help stop symptoms, disorders, and disease.

VITAMIN C

When you think of one antioxidant in particular, vitamin C, you probably don't think of celery. Whatever small amount of vitamin C it contains can't really add up to anything, can it? Quite the contrary. The vitamin C in celery is more remarkable than that in a tomato. It's more remarkable than the vitamin C in broccoli. It's even more remarkable than the vitamin C in an orange. That's because celery's unique variety of vitamin C requires no methylation in the liver for the body to be able to use it. This means that the vitamin C in celery juice can boost the immune system unlike any other vitamin C because of this bioavailable, pre-methylated form.

Most anyone with most any symptom, condition, or illness is dealing with a sick liver, one that's stagnant and sluggish and full of toxins and pathogens: viruses, bacteria, toxic heavy metals, pesticides, herbicides, old DDT, and even traces of radiation, among other troublemakers. Not to mention that we unknowingly bombard our livers with high-fat diets, whether full of healthy or unhealthy fats, on a daily basis. Usually, nutrient methylation takes place inside the liver; medical research and science don't know the degree to which the liver is responsible for this conversion process, making vitamins and minerals usable for the rest of the body once they leave this organ. Put together the overburdened, compromised livers that so many are dealing with and this critical function the liver is meant to perform, and you've got widespread methylation issues. This means that while the vitamin C someone receives from a given food will be helpful, the liver will still have to process it—yet one more task on its endless to-do list, one it probably can't fulfill to its highest degree.

With the vitamin C in celery juice, the liver doesn't need to process, conform, convert, and methylate it to make it useful and usable for the body. It's pre-methylated to the fullest extent. While the vitamin C from other fruits and vegetables is important, to say the least, the vitamin C from celery juice stands alone in this way. It's part of why you start to heal from celery juice.

This vitamin C has a special relationship with celery juice's sodium cluster salts, too. Because cluster salts have an ability to surround the other nutrients in celery juice and help deliver them throughout the body, they're able to attach themselves to vitamin C and travel with it to wherever the immune system needs these two components most.

More is better when it comes to celery juice's vitamin C. What seems like celery's small serving of vitamin C is actually much larger when you think about drinking the juice from one whole bunch of it. Concentrating that pre-methylated vitamin C from an entire celery head into a 16-ounce glass and drinking it on an empty stomach means you're getting an instant immune system boost.

People who suffer with autoimmune issues—meaning that they have high viral or even bacterial loads—tend to have more difficulty detoxifying because their livers are overloaded and stagnant, which means the blood consistently fills up with toxins, particularly viral debris. Blood that's saturated with neurotoxins, dermatoxins, and other viral waste matter can lead to diagnoses ranging from multiple sclerosis (MS) all the way to Lyme disease (although this is not because doctors or blood labs know that tests are picking up on viral byproduct, and that these conditions are really viral; tests detect them only as unidentified inflammation markers). Usually in these cases where someone is highly viral, vitamin C is not easy to process, especially in high quantities. The vitamin C in celery juice is different: it's gentle, bioavailable, and easier on someone who is compromised in any way. It leaves the body easily, too, and as it leaves, celery juice's vitamin C assists people by both binding onto viral waste matter in the bloodstream and escorting it out of the body through the kidneys and even the skin. That is, it helps eliminate the viral debris that otherwise causes autoimmune conditions to worsen constantly. Celery juice's vitamin C is an answer and an antidote for people who are struggling with symptoms and conditions caused by viral culprits.

PREBIOTIC FACTOR

Other prebiotic foods starve unproductive bacteria, hindering their ability to fuel themselves at least for that moment, which in turn allows colonies of good bacteria to thrive. Celery juice's prebiotic factor works on another level that other prebiotics don't. It not only starves unproductive bacteria; it actively breaks down, weakens, and destroys unproductive bacteria.

Celery juice also takes away food sources from these bugs in the gut. Colonies of unproductive bacteria survive in part on little storage bins of food rotting in the digestive tract. These tucked-away pockets are like their rations for hard times. Celery juice is like a grenade thrown into these pockets, breaking up old buildup of dehydrated fats and proteins and dispersing them. Any unproductive bacteria that survive celery juice's initial bacterial die-off effect end up losing their food source. That's the cleansing power of sodium cluster salts.

And here's a feat that no other herb, fruit, vegetable, or other prebiotic can perform: Celery juice prepares the broken-down, dead bacteria as food for productive bacteria in the gut. As the bad bacteria become saturated with sodium cluster salts, they can actually be devoured by good bacteria. The reason this works is that celery juice's sodium cluster salts disinfect unproductive bacteria, drawing out their poisons after destroying them. The bacterial cells become empty, tasty carcasses for good bacteria to consume and prosper.

HYDROBIOACTIVE WATER

You'll hear some sources say that celery juice is mostly water. That misses one of the most critical understandings about this humble herb and what it does for our bodies. Yes, celery juice has what we could easily call water. It's not the water you would fill a swimming pool with, though. It's not the water you'd put in a fish pond. It's not the water that comes out of a hose or your faucet or that falls from the sky as rain. There's not a stream on earth that would flow with the water in celery juice. It's simply not water in the way we think of water. Celery juice is a living, breathing drink. The water in celery juice holds life in it in a special way. It's *hydrobioactive water.*

Celery juice and plain water are so different that it's not a good idea to mix them. This is why I advise against diluting celery juice with water or adding ice cubes to it. Regular water renders celery juice's benefits useless. It's also why I advise against dehydrating celery or celery juice and then reconstituting it with water. That doesn't re-create a glass of celery juice, because regular water isn't living. Freshly juiced celery's liquid sustains life—and therefore sustains your life. Saying that it's no different from water is undermining celery juice. It's like saying to your daughter that her school project isn't special; it's the same as everyone else's. You would never say that. Her school project is entirely different from the rest of the class's. It's signature.

Which is why when we hear rumors that drinking a glass of water is basically the same as drinking a glass of celery juice, we don't need to get on that doubt train. Celery juice is a healing liquid, a structured tonic that's filled with the life of the herb and that plant's life story, energy, and nutrients. We shouldn't insult celery juice, as though that celery plant did nothing to transform the water it took in when it was growing. We shouldn't worry that celery juice is nothing more than a glass of water with a few nutrients floating in it.

A glass of celery juice is saturated with information. It's saturated with intelligence. It's saturated with ample amounts of trace minerals and sodium cluster salts. It's not even just that, though. The hydrobioactive water in celery juice is organized in such a way that it uniquely suspends those life-giving nutrients and phytochemical compounds so that they're ready to be delivered to your body. This water is alive and has a system to it, one that will be studied in the years to come.

The water that's inside your blood is different from the drinking water we pour into a glass, too. The water in your blood is an organized part of your life force. As part of your blood, it's not just water anymore. That's how celery juice is. We have to see the water content of celery juice as the life force of the celery plant, just as our blood is the life force of us. That life force from celery juice is made to mix with our life force, our blood, and become one. Because we're living organisms, if we consume this living water, it's more beneficial to us than consuming regular water. The hydrobioactive water in celery juice even goes beyond living water. It's life.

"This chapter bears witness to you. Your suffering is real, you don't deserve it, and your body hasn't let you down. With the proper information, you can heal."

— Anthony William, Medical Medium

CHAPTER 3

Relief from Your Symptoms and Conditions

What you will find in this chapter is advanced healing information about why people suffer and how they can finally find relief.

Labels for symptoms, conditions, illnesses, disorders, and diseases—especially chronic ones—don't always tell you too much about the cause behind the health struggle. That's often because the cause remains unknown and theoretical as medical research and science continue to look for answers. It is such a trying experience to struggle with your health. On top of the physical or mental challenge, there's the emotional trial of losing trust in your body and facing people who don't understand your suffering, who make light of it or even call it into question. There are so many conflicting, confusing messages that can make people wonder if they somehow deserve their illness or if they've conjured it with negative thoughts or made it up to get attention. Here's the truth: it takes so much

strength to weather the isolation and disrespect while continuing to look for answers and solve the mystery. This chapter aims to clear up the mystery and offer validation for the very real causes and experiences of chronic illness, however briefly this short space allows, while also providing insights into how celery juice can help alleviate or prevent your particular health concern. This chapter bears witness to you. Your suffering is real, you don't deserve it, and your body hasn't let you down. With the proper information, you can heal.

Many of you reading this will be unaware of the Medical Medium series's work to demystify chronic and mystery illness. Know that by this point, thousands of doctors across this country alone, never mind globally, are using the Medical Medium books in their offices as reference guides to help their patients. This started because over the years, patients brought the books to their doctors' appointments, talked about their improvements, and asked their doctors to incorporate the books' information into their own guidance. For many years before the publication of these books, too, I worked alongside doctors in their practices, providing advanced medical information to assist them in helping patients who were suffering from chronic and mystery illnesses.

If your main health struggle is not in this chapter's list, don't despair. I wish I had room to include everyone here. You'll find more symptom and condition causes explained, and often in more detail, in the other Medical Medium books, along with guidance on how to recover. Also, just because your issue is not in this chapter, that does not mean celery juice can't be helpful for you. Keep reading. You're likely to find at least one symptom you've experienced in this list, and addressing it will put you on the road to better overall health.

Now for the main event. You're about to get a window into the true causes of about 100 symptoms and conditions, all told. Much of it could be surprising if you're used to hearing "idiopathic" or "cause unknown" and never really understanding why your joints hurt or your mother was flattened with fatigue for part of your childhood or your sister had trouble conceiving or your uncle is suffering from tinnitus or your cousin has multiple autoimmune diagnoses or your nephew has trouble sleeping at night. In each case, I'll also show how celery juice can address what's ailing a person to allow you and your family to recover and return to better health.

ADDICTION

Often addiction is spurred by a lack of nutrients. A dysfunctional liver that's not able to transform nutrients and deliver them adequately through the bloodstream to the brain and the rest of the body is one major part of addiction. A high level of toxic heavy metals such as mercury, copper, and aluminum in the liver and brain is another major part of it. Emotional duress, stress, compromises, wounds, and injuries can also contribute. Celery juice can help with all of it.

Celery juice stabilizes all aspects of the liver, including glucose reception. Here's a big reason why that's important: most people who struggle with addictive actions are also dealing with insulin resistance. Celery juice helps alleviate insulin resistance and helps cells open up and receive glucose without having to lean on insulin alone.

Celery juice nourishes the brain, restoring neurons and replenishing neurotransmitters. It helps neutralize, disarm, and release toxic heavy metals from the brain, also helping flush the byproduct that results when metals collide and interact with each other. Celery juice's plant hormones also help protect brain cells—slowing down the death of brain cells and even assisting with the production of new cells—so that someone suffering through emotional trials can find balance and calm. Further, the plant hormones from celery juice improve, strengthen, and reinvigorate the adrenals, balancing them when they're over- or underactive to counteract addictive behavior.

Another benefit of celery juice is that it alkalizes the bloodstream and body, reducing acidosis, which can minimize addictive impulses all on its own, reducing that feeling of needing to reach for a cigarette or another piece of chocolate. Celery juice helps flush out of people's systems old drugs and other pharmaceuticals that are involved in so much addictive suffering—it helps flush them out of the liver and bloodstream, which leads to fewer addictive relapses.

ADRENAL COMPLICATIONS

Adrenal Fatigue, Stress, Weakness, and Disease

Celery juice helps address any kind of adrenal dysfunction by restoring damaged adrenal tissue and weakened adrenal glands, whether they've been affected by disease or by a state of constant, chronic fight-or-flight. Medical research and science are unaware of just how much our adrenals do for us and the dozens of diverse, complex blends of hormones they produce that support everything we do in life. Our adrenals are the ultimate hormone producers, more so even than our reproductive systems. Whether we're experiencing a hardship; experiencing love, joy, and happiness; performing simple tasks like going to the bathroom, showering, brushing our teeth, or consuming and digesting food; or anything in between, the adrenals are there, producing a unique adrenaline blend to help us function.

We have two adrenals, a right and a left. Each of our two adrenals produces different varieties of hormones. Usually, they aren't the same strength—one has become weaker than the other from overwork, so it produces less adrenaline, forcing the other to then overwork and eventually weaken as well. Components of celery juice have the ability to enter the adrenals and saturate adrenal tissue, strengthening every aspect of the adrenal cells—healing, pampering, and coddling them. I should probably give sodium cluster salts the nickname "sodium glandular salts" because of how powerful they are for restoring the adrenals. Sodium cluster salts are a miracle for the adrenal glands. Sea salt and mountain rock salt are often heralded as good for us—we look up to them as being the best. And yes, those are higher quality salts. Still, their variety of sodium does not serve as a medicinal; those salts do not offer what celery juice's sodium cluster salts do. Trace minerals are bonded to celery juice's cluster salts in a way we don't see with any other variety of food or salt. Cluster salts reestablish and ignite life in adrenal cells, also allowing the glands to rapidly produce new cells that are healthy and strong.

Celery juice balances the adrenal glands so that the weaker one can catch up to the stronger one—and allows the two glands to communicate with each other, a facet of their function that medical research and science have not yet discovered. Celery juice's very powerful electrolytes are what create this inter-gland communication: celery juice's mineral salts enter one adrenal gland, exit through the bloodstream, and enter the other gland with information that it carried from the first adrenal.

For more on adrenal fatigue, see the section on "Fatigue" in this chapter, as well as the full chapter on the subject in *Medical Medium*. There, you'll also find information on the 56 unique adrenaline blends that provide for our needs on a daily basis. Celery juice is such a blessing to help restore our adrenals so that we don't become or stay susceptible to adrenal complications, dysfunction, and disease.

ALZHEIMER'S DISEASE, DEMENTIA, AND MEMORY ISSUES

Memory issues can occur in many different ways, whether in the form of trouble retrieving long-term memories, losing short-term memories, or even fluctuations, where short-term and long-term memory issues flip back and forth. We're talking about more than those days when you're really busy and you're misplacing your belongings, maybe even forgetting where you parked at a busy shopping center—although celery juice helps, too, with that kind of task overload, where you're trying to remember a dozen things in the midst of an overly stressful day. When we talk about serious memory issues such as Alzheimer's disease and dementia, what we're talking about without realizing it are toxic heavy metals in the brain, the most common being mercury and aluminum, with close

runners-up of copper, nickel, cadmium, lead, and arsenic. Everybody has a different volume of toxic heavy metals in the brain in different combinations, with some metals directly crossing each other's paths, some metals touching each other side by side, and some metals in blended alloys.

Specifically, memory issues occur when those metals oxidize. Oxidizing metals lead to discharge. Think of a patch of metal rusting on a car, becoming crusty and bubbling up. This is essentially what happens in the brain, albeit on a microscopic or even nanoscopic scale. One major cause of this oxidative reaction is a high level of fat in the bloodstream—from healthy fats *or* unhealthy fats. Whether the diet is filled with high-quality oils, nuts, seeds, avocados, cheese, eggs, chicken, fish, and beef or hydrogenated oils, cakes, cookies, doughnuts, and other fried foods, the resulting fat in the bloodstream leads to this oxidative reaction with toxic heavy metals in the brain. The toxic heavy metals start to break down, and not in a positive manner. They rust, change form and shape, rupture, or even grow and expand as they run together. Celery juice, as the most powerful electrolyte source on the planet—nothing can surpass it or even equal it—helps repair the damage.

For one thing, celery juice's complex blend of trace minerals not only helps restore neurotransmitter chemicals; the blend also offers complete neurotransmitter chemicals, which is critical because rusting metals' oxidative runoff clouds up neurotransmitters, making them dirty and less useful. For another, celery juice cleans off the oxidative runoff of toxic heavy metals from neurons, another essential function since neurons can't sustain themselves while being bombarded by heavy metal runoff. Celery juice binds onto the oxidative material, neutralizing it and making it less toxic. And by reviving haggard, injured neurotransmitters that are sitting on neurons as well as offering complete neurotransmitter chemicals, celery juice starts to help improve memory and can even help reverse Alzheimer's disease.

If you think you haven't been exposed to toxic heavy metals, think again. Have you ever eaten a can of tuna? Consumed a beverage from an aluminum can? Eaten a snack or sandwich that was wrapped or cooked in aluminum foil? Have you ever had a drink of water that wasn't the purest, perhaps some of the tap water that's served at millions of restaurants worldwide? Have you ever taken a pharmaceutical? These everyday sources bring heavy metals into our bodies. Yes, even pharmaceuticals contain heavy metals. There are even traces of toxic heavy metals in the air that we breathe in, from sources such as exhaust fumes and jet fuel. Plus, we inherit metals that are passed down from generation to generation, with mercury and copper the most common. Depression can be a symptom of toxic heavy metals in the brain. So can anxiety. The effects of those metals can show themselves very quickly in some people—oxidative stress can even happen to young adults—and sometimes it takes longer, developing over years. It

depends on where in the brain the metals reside, how long they've been there, and how much they're oxidizing. And when those heavy metals lead to memory issues, what everyone who's suffering in this situation has in common is that the metals are breaking down, changing in formation, oxidizing, running into and saturating adjacent brain tissue, and affecting neurons and neurotransmitter chemicals. When neurotransmitters are diminished and weakened, brain fog can also be a factor, whether before or after the onset of memory loss.

Given the seriousness of dementia, Alzheimer's, and other memory loss conditions, a 2-ounce shot of celery juice a week is not going to help the problem. Look for tips in the next chapter on healing advanced conditions by consuming larger quantities of celery juice, and read up on the Heavy Metal Detox Smoothie in Chapter 8.

AMYOTROPHIC LATERAL SCLEROSIS (ALS, LOU GEHRIG'S DISEASE)

ALS is still a medical mystery. It's not diagnosed alongside an actual, underlying "find" to explain what is occurring in the body. A multitude of neurological symptoms can occur for someone living with an ALS diagnosis—and in truth, diagnoses are often a result of a doctor eye-witnessing symptoms, because it is such a mystery.

The true cause of ALS is a viral infection inside the brain, most commonly HHV-6 accompanying another virus or two (for instance, shingles or EBV) in other areas of the body. Viral neurotoxins are what cause the symptoms of ALS, and these particular neurotoxins can only be created when there's a large amount of toxic heavy metals present in the system: aluminum at the highest level, mercury at the second-highest level, and copper at the third. Reactions among these metals lead to corrosion, and this can put a strain on neurons. Corrosive heavy metal deposits are also easy food for HHV-6, because they often reside in the brain, too. And when toxic heavy metals and their corrosive deposits are present in other parts of the body, they provide fuel for nearby herpetic viruses involved in the disease.

Most people with ALS are hurting everywhere. They are often struggling in many ways, with a variety of deficiencies and chronic inflammation throughout the entire body. Their livers are never functioning well, and that can mean trouble converting nutrients, which is what causes the deficiencies. Celery juice is so bioavailable, with most of its nutrients (such as its unique vitamin C) and chemical compounds needing no conversion in the liver. This is a godsend for those suffering with ALS, as it means they can access the healing properties the juice has to offer.

ALS symptoms can improve and neuron regeneration can take place with a strong antiviral protocol and the proper toxic heavy metal cleanse. For guidance on both, check out *Thyroid Healing*. Celery juice is another tool to help this occur faster. In ALS, neurons need to be replenished rapidly, and celery juice is the best electrolyte there is for this. Its sodium cluster salts and the trace minerals connected to them—along with antioxidants, bioavailable vitamin C, and other nutrients that cluster salts deliver with ease thanks to their unique velocity—not only replenish neurons, they boost and protect adjacent brain tissue. Not to mention that with sodium cluster salts, celery juice offers neurotransmitter chemicals in complete form. This gives someone with injured neurons, as is the case in ALS, a chance to heal. Increasing celery juice to 32 ounces daily, coupled with a daily Heavy Metal Detox Smoothie, which you'll read about in Chapter 8, and other supports that I recommend in *Thyroid Healing* and *Medical Medium*, is a wise choice for those suffering with ALS symptoms.

AUTOIMMUNE CONDITIONS

If you're struggling with a health problem that's been labeled as autoimmune, it is not the result of your body attacking itself. It is your body going after pathogens. The autoimmune theory took off in the 1950s with no science to prove it, and it still has no scientific support. Yes, autoimmune conditions are serious. Anything labeled autoimmune is serious. These are real symptoms and real illnesses, and people really are suffering. The term *autoimmune*, though, is a misnomer. If medical research and science were advanced enough when these conditions started to take hold of the population years ago, they would have used the term *viral immune* instead, because the body is going after invaders, most often viruses.

It's not doctors' fault that they tell patients their bodies are attacking themselves. They get stuck in the autoimmune trap. Medical school does not teach physicians what's really responsible for hundreds of conditions, because these remain scientific mysteries. Since researchers can't detect what's really wrong, they conclude it must be someone's own immune system destroying their organs, glands, or tissue. The most reasonable explanation seems to be that someone's body must be at fault. If this were true, it would be important to disclose to the patient. It's not what's really going on, though, and hearing that your body has turned on you is detrimental to the healing process.

That's especially true for the younger people receiving autoimmune diagnoses today. The younger you are, the more that message that your body is faulty or destroying itself gets cemented in your sense of self. Hearing, too, that your autoimmune condition is genetic (which isn't true, either) is a difficult combination. When a young woman walks out of the doctor's office with a brand-new diagnosis of Hashimoto's thyroiditis and the message that her immune system is destroying her thyroid, and that this dysfunction is encoded in the very fiber of her being, recovering from the emotional blow of this mental image adds a whole other level of needed healing on top of getting better from the condition itself.

There's nothing comforting about an autoimmune diagnosis. The only consolation comes from having your suffering seen, recognized, and given a name. If only medical research and science weren't baffled by chronic illness and they could tell you: Yes, your suffering is real. What is truly occurring is your body creating antibodies to seek out and destroy pathogens. That is, your immune system is going after a bug. These bugs are so elusive. There are hundreds of varieties of common, everyday viruses, and new mutations appear every year. They wreak havoc in people's organs and the rest of their bodies, creating a range of autoimmune diagnoses because doctors detect inflammation that they can't explain.

In cases where researchers think they've identified autoantibodies, meaning antibodies created by your immune system to go after your own body, they're mistaken. They are real antibodies produced by your immune system. They are not produced to attack you, though. They're produced to attack a virus. Usually, it's a virus buried too deep in your system for current medical testing to detect.

In truth, it's those undetected pathogens creating inflammation. It's not a misfire of the immune system. Nor is it caused by foods that are considered inflammatory. The reason that certain foods lead to inflammation is that they feed the pathogens, and it's the prospering pathogens themselves that create inflammation. Our immune system's job is to look out for viruses and bacteria and destroy them. When we have a lowered immune system, that's a difficult task. Even a lowered immune system doesn't mean it turns on the body and starts attacking itself, though. There's always a hidden pathogen.

Anyone suffering with any sort of condition labeled autoimmune is struggling with endocrine system issues as a result. The plant hormones that only celery juice possesses are critical for helping remedy this. These plant hormones enter into every endocrine gland to help support, strengthen, and balance them so they can come out of a hypo or hyper state. This leveling of the endocrine glands, from the adrenals to the pancreas, allows them to produce the proper levels of hormones.

As we established, everyone suffering with an autoimmune condition is also suffering with a viral infection. Some are chronic, low-grade infections from a virus such as Epstein-Barr, and some are more severe infections from a virus such as HHV-6. Some people are struggling with trigeminal neuralgia caused by the shingles virus. Some are suffering with multiple sclerosis caused by EBV. (There used to be just a handful of illnesses deemed to be autoimmune. Now dozens are on the list. This will keep going, so that at some point nearly every condition that's not understood by medical research and science will be tagged as autoimmune and genetic, without proof to back that up.) In all of these situations and more, celery juice's sodium cluster salts are the ultimate virus destroyers.

This is why people see their inflammation reduce when they're on celery juice. Since inflammation is caused by viruses, when cluster salts destroy viral cells' outer membranes, weakening the cells and driving down their numbers, mysterious inflammation goes down, too. On top of this, cluster salts bind onto the waste matter such as neurotoxins that viruses produce when they feed on toxins such as toxic heavy metals. Viral neurotoxins are another aspect of autoimmune illnesses of which medical research and science are unaware. In reality, they inflame the nervous systems of everyone dealing with autoimmune symptoms. Celery juice's cluster salts kill off their cause—a viral load—while defusing neurotoxin waste frees up the nervous system so that people can get their lives back.

It's this potent combination of celery juice's plant hormones and sodium cluster salts that we can thank for helping people recover from the symptoms that medicine calls autoimmune disease. We're also going to look more specifically at what medical research and science don't realize really causes some of the most common autoimmune issues, along with how celery juice can help. Keep in mind that depending on how pronounced your situation is, you may need to incorporate other healing information from the Medical Medium series along with your celery juice.

Fibromyalgia

Celery juice is very helpful for fibromyalgia because it defuses the toxins responsible for the condition: Epstein-Barr viral neurotoxins. These neurotoxins landing on nerves are responsible for the peripheral and central nerve inflammation that fibro sufferers experience. When celery juice comes into the system, its sodium cluster salts attach themselves to the neurotoxins and carry them out of the body safely so that nerves are less exposed to the EBV neurotoxins. It goes beyond that, too. Often people with fibro have highly toxic livers that go undiagnosed. Celery juice cleanses and purifies the liver, removing many of the neurotoxin poisons that the virus produces in the organ before they even get a chance to reach nerves throughout the body. With use of celery juice over time, overall body pain can reduce and particular "hot spots" that fibro sufferers deal with can improve substantially.

Lyme Disease

Celery juice destroys bacteria such as *Borrelia*, *Bartonella*, and *Babesia*. If you believe you have a bacterial infection, then celery juice is the right tool.

That said, you may be interested to know that Lyme disease is a chronic *viral* infection. While you might have been diagnosed with a bacterial infection, the symptoms of Lyme are viral. Even if bacteria such as *Borrelia* are present, they're not causing what makes Lyme patients suffer. The symptoms of Lyme are neurological, and bacteria don't create neurological symptoms because they don't produce neurotoxins. Only viruses feeding on toxic heavy metals such as mercury, aluminum, and copper—as well as gluten, eggs, dairy, pesticides, herbicides, and fungicides that are inside our livers and other parts of our bodies—create the neurotoxins that cause Lyme disease.

Specifically, only viruses from the herpetic family are at work here: EBV and its over 60 undiscovered mutations and strains; all the varieties of shingles, including unknown strains that don't cause any visible rash or pustules; and multiple mutations of HHV-6, HHV-7, and the undiscovered HHV-10 through HHV-16. These viruses release neurotoxins that inflame the entire nervous system, causing the neurological symptoms of Lyme disease. This is why many with Lyme also eventually receive diagnoses of other chronic conditions such as MS, rheumatoid arthritis (RA), Hashimoto's thyroiditis, fibromyalgia, and myalgic encephalomyelitis/chronic fatigue syndrome (ME/CFS). These and more are EBV-caused. So is Lyme. They all come from the same source.

Doctors don't realize this. They're taught that if anything, some of the conditions are EBV-*related*. They don't know it's the undiscovered cause of all of it. So with diagnosis, the lines are blurred and mistakes are made. What you need to know is the truth: that the myriad neurological symptoms that Lyme sufferers experience are caused by chronic low-grade viral infections, with viruses feeding off the foods they like and releasing neurotoxins.

If you're still attached to the past and the old ways of thinking about Lyme, then as I said, celery juice is still your go-to, because it eradicates *Borrelia*, *Bartonella*, *Babesia*, and any new bacteria that medical research and science try to pin on Lyme disease in their confusion. Don't let your or your doctor's disbelief that Lyme is viral discredit celery juice. It's a potent antibacterial. It will still help you. By the way, as I mentioned earlier, since the Medical Medium books have been published, doctors have started to use them as guidelines in their practices. Doctors have been particularly interested in Lyme disease guidance. That Lyme disease is viral makes more sense to them than the bacterial theories. There are now thousands of doctors who support this information. Celery juice will also help if this advanced future information about Lyme disease— that it's viral—resonates with you. As you read in the autoimmune introduction, celery juice is a potent antiviral.

Multiple Sclerosis (MS)

Celery juice can be a great source of healing when you're dealing with multiple sclerosis. You can receive powerful healing benefits from it for a number of reasons. The true cause of MS is EBV releasing neurotoxins and inflaming the central nervous system. The sodium cluster salts in celery juice hinder and deter the virus, weakening it and breaking it down by dissolving the outer membranes of the viral cells. Once the viral load has been reduced, MS patients can find reprieve and relief as their symptoms start to disappear.

Celery juice also detoxifies the toxins that someone with MS is harboring. People with MS struggle with stagnant, sluggish livers that are filled with viral toxins and debris as well as toxic heavy metals and other liver troublemakers. Celery juice helps cleanse the liver, neutralizing and binding onto these toxins and neurotoxins and then escorting them out of the body.

All of this viral and toxin cleansing reduces inflammation, one of the main symptoms that MS sufferers encounter. That could be short-term or long-term inflammation of the myelin nerve sheaths or joints. Celery juice provides relief from both.

People with MS have imbalanced endocrine systems, too, and the plant hormones that celery juice offers to help re-strengthen the endocrine glands are invaluable. Also, celery juice's unique variety of bioavailable, assimilable vitamin C is instantly usable for the body. With most any nutrient, the liver must convert it. The vitamin C in celery juice needs no conversion. It's already ready to give the immune system a boost. That means everything for someone living with MS—someone who's up against the Epstein-Barr virus and needs this powerful immune support.

Celery juice alone is one of the most powerful tools for coping with MS. When combined with other truths about MS and how to work on healing it, truths found in the Medical Medium series, people living with MS can truly be on their way to freeing themselves from the various symptoms associated with the disease.

Myalgic Encephalomyelitis/Chronic Fatigue Syndrome (ME/CFS), Chronic Fatigue Immune Dysfunction Syndrome (CFIDS), Systemic Exertion Intolerance Disease (SEID)

Some of the newer terms for chronic fatigue syndrome got their names from medical research and science finally recognizing that when people complained about being chronically tired, feeling like their legs were bags of cement, being unable to keep their eyes open and also unable to sleep, and suffering from a host of other symptoms that made it a struggle to function day to day, it was real. As medical communities started to take these complaints seriously, they realized that brain inflammation could be a factor, which is how terms such as *encephalomyelitis* (brain and spinal cord inflammation) became involved.

Long before the medical establishment recognized CFS, I saw it as an actual illness and described it as *neurological fatigue*. As I've always said, Epstein-Barr virus is the cause. This is true for the millions of people around the world suffering from it. More pronounced cases of ME/CFS are caused by certain strains of EBV that are a little more aggressive and create stronger neurotoxins that inflame the entire nervous system. Neurons in the brain are even affected, causing brain fog, confusion, and difficulty walking with any vigor.

As with any viral infection, celery juice is our best weapon. EBV cannot become immune to celery juice's sodium cluster salts. Further, people dealing with ME/CFS have compromised immune systems, and white blood cells find peace and solace with the trace minerals that celery juice offers. Its vitamin C also fuels the immune system so it can seek out and destroy the EBV that causes ME/CFS.

You'll find that most everyone with ME/CFS these days is also diagnosed with Lyme disease. See the connection? EBV is behind both of them and always has been. They're mistakenly diagnosed as two separate problems, even though you know now they come from the same source. Celery juice has a profound effect on recovering someone's nervous system when it's been compromised and inflamed from EBV, and that makes all the difference whether someone is trying to heal from ME/CFS, Lyme, or both.

Rheumatoid Arthritis (RA), Psoriatic Arthritis (PsA), and Scleroderma

These types of joint pain are viral inflammation caused by EBV. The reason that RA and PsA are mistaken for the immune system attacking someone's joints is that medical research has identified antibodies present that it believes to be autoantibodies. Again, in truth, those antibodies aren't a misfire of the immune system. EBV is what's causing the inflammation of joints and nerves. The antibodies are created by your immune system to go after the virus, not to attack your body. Celery juice steps in to help out, as it is extremely antiviral, helping rid the body of EBV and alleviate symptoms of RA and PsA.

By the way, PsA is not caused by calcium stones. It is caused by EBV sitting inside the liver, feeding off copper and mercury and releasing neurotoxins into the bloodstream that then settle in joint areas. In this case, EBV is also releasing dermatoxins, which surface in the skin around joints, causing bouts of rashes. PsA can take many different forms depending on how toxic someone's liver is and how viral they are. Celery juice helps eliminate the copper and mercury culprits from the liver; that alone brings down the viral load, since these toxic heavy metals are favored foods for the virus. At the same time, celery juice's sodium cluster salts help rid pockets of EBV throughout the body so someone can finally move forward with healing.

With scleroderma, dermatoxins and neurotoxins are present from an EBV strain feeding on mercury and copper. In particular, insecticides, other pesticides, and fungicides provide viral fuel here. The resulting dermatoxins create heat and deep tissue pain. Celery juice's cleansing action inside the liver helps neutralize the pesticides, fungicides, and herbicides and flush them from the body. Celery juice helps cleanse the liver of dermatoxins, too, so that someone with scleroderma can eventually get relief from symptoms.

AUTOIMMUNE SKIN CONDITIONS

Dermatitis

There's a variety of dermatitis that I call *classic dermatitis*, in which a common garden variety of EBV feeds on deposits of aluminum, copper, and pesticides inside the liver, causing dry skin, dandruff, or patchy, irritated skin. Celery juice helps destroy the low-grade viral infection of EBV, also helping dislodge and remove old pesticides such as DDT while neutralizing aluminum and copper byproduct.

Seborrheic dermatitis is more the result of a pre-fatty or fatty liver, leading someone to develop thick, dirty blood. In this case, there's not a virus involved. It's a liver filled with a little bit of everything, with toxins escaping the liver and making it to the skin instead of being stored back in the liver or sent out of the body. Celery juice revives the liver, flushing out the overload of toxins and reinvigorating liver cells so that the organ can perform its over 2,000 chemical functions, many of them undiscovered by medical research and science. One important function is for the liver to deliver nutrients to other organs such as the skin—this alone helps reduce seborrheic dermatitis.

Eczema, Psoriasis, Rosacea, and Actinic Keratosis

Eczema and psoriasis are caused by a low-grade infection of a herpetic virus inside the liver. Most commonly, that virus is EBV. When the virus feeds off toxic copper and mercury that are also in the liver and then excretes them, that copper turns into a dermatoxin. These dermatoxins build up and exit the liver, eventually finding their way to the lower levels of the dermis. Once there, the body tries to detox them by pushing the dermatoxins up through the skin. This can lead to almost 100 varieties of rashes that are deemed to be eczema or psoriasis or are given different names. In none of these cases is the immune system attacking the skin. That's an inaccurate explanation that comes out of misunderstanding how eczema and psoriasis really work.

Because celery juice feeds the skin, people who drink it experience amazing skin benefits. This includes watching eczema and psoriasis disappear over time. Celery juice's coumarins surface through the skin, reinvigorating skin cells from deep within. (More on coumarins in Chapter 7.) This results in less skin cell death and deterioration and supports nerves, blood vessels, and blood flow through the skin. The special variety of vitamin C in celery juice helps restore the liver's personalized immune system to help fight off any viral load that's present.

Rosacea is a particular form of eczema that can appear in many forms on the face and neck. Celery juice helps by flushing out the mercury-based toxins that reside in the small intestinal tract and feed EBV that's also there. Once celery juice's sodium cluster salts minimize the viral load inside the intestines and help disarm and neutralize the mercury toxins and byproduct present, rosacea can start to clear up. Eliminating foods such as eggs, dairy, and gluten that feed EBV can speed up the process.

Actinic keratosis is another form of eczema. This time, it's a low-grade viral infection feeding on mercury and some copper. Celery juice helps the same way it helps rosacea and eczema, by helping rid you of metals and destroying the hidden virus.

People with more advanced, aggressive cases of eczema and psoriasis usually have a higher toxic heavy metal load and viral load inside the liver. When they first start drinking celery juice and it begins to flush out the liver, it starts to move around the toxic heavy metals and fight the virus, and a large viral die-off can result. This die-off can release more dermatoxins into the system than normal, leading to what seems like an elevated outbreak of eczema and psoriasis. If this happens to you, know that it's a temporary healing reaction. Lower the amount of celery juice you drink and give it some time. Celery juice is your best friend for eventually alleviating your skin condition. In the meantime, turn to Chapter 8, "More Healing Guidance," and research the rest of the Medical Medium series to learn about what else you can do to help your skin.

People often look for health advice far and wide, trying some that may not be all that helpful. Many times when people start a new routine such as celery juice, they start other initiatives, too. They may begin a new diet at the same time, for example—one that isn't in line with what they really need. Because they also just started celery juice, it often gets the blame. Keep this in mind if you are having what seems like a reaction to celery juice. Did you also start following health advice from another source around the same time you started celery juice? It could be that you're consuming foods that feed the virus, and that's the real reason for your outbreak, rather than a large viral die-off or detoxifying liver. If you start avoiding unproductive foods as well (see Chapter 8), you'll help along your healing.

Lichen Sclerosus

This skin condition comes from a combination of copper, mercury, and old, inherited DDT along with a low-grade viral infection. Celery juice can help loosen, remove, and rid old deposits of DDT and toxic heavy metals from inside the liver at the same time it reduces the viral load, giving people with lichen sclerosus relief when they use celery juice long term.

Lupus-Style Rashes

This type of rash is caused by EBV feeding off mercury and aluminum, creating a dermatoxin that surfaces to the skin in areas where important lymphatic highways reside. It's why butterfly-shaped rashes can appear on the face, along with other forms of rashes that can land somebody a diagnosis of lupus. Once again, this is not the body attacking itself. It is a low-grade viral infection. Many people with lupus also get diagnosed separately with EBV because the doctor sees EBV come through in a blood

test. Usually, they still won't associate the virus with the lupus-style rashes. If a lupus patient visits a Lyme doctor, they may end up with a Lyme diagnosis as well—still not realizing that it all traces back to the same source: EBV. Celery juice helps with all of it. The sodium cluster salts reduce the underlying viral infection and help defuse and neutralize the dermatoxins responsible for the rash itself.

Vitiligo

Celery juice can help people struggling with vitiligo because it disarms the aluminum byproduct that floats around in the bloodstream, creating this condition. Medical research and science are unaware that vitiligo is caused by a virus such as HHV-6 or EBV feeding on aluminum and traces of formaldehyde in the liver and elsewhere in the body, releasing an aluminum-based dermatoxin that, when it enters the skin, destroys the melanin pigments inside skin cells. This is what leads to the white spots and other discolorations that occur for someone living with vitiligo. It is not the skin's immune system attacking the skin pigment. It is a real illness with a real cause. Celery juice helps by going after the virus responsible as well as helping flush out the aluminum and traces of formaldehyde that have built up in the liver and other parts of the body.

BALANCE ISSUES

Vertigo, Ménière's Disease, and Dizziness

People suffer with so many different varieties of balance issues. Some people experience severe symptoms, where they feel the room spin, and for others it's a little milder, with more of a sense that they're on a rocking boat, with the floor beneath them moving. If there's no obvious cause such as an injury, concussion, or brain tumor, this is all a mystery to medical research and science. In truth, the vagus nerve has everything to do with unexplained balance struggles.

The vagus nerve, which is actually a pair of cranial nerves, runs from the brain stem down through the neck and chest and into the abdomen. It's a very sensitive nerve. Viral neurotoxins from the Epstein-Barr virus are some of its greatest enemies and irritants. When EBV is active in the body, the neurotoxins that the virus releases can attach themselves to the vagus nerve and cause it to swell. The degree of swelling can vary along the nerve. Sometimes it's only the tip of the nerve that's swollen, down near the stomach, where it branches off. Sometimes it's swollen higher up, in the chest, which can result in tightness and trouble breathing that's hard to understand since a pulmonologist has given a stamp of approval, saying there's nothing wrong with the lungs. For some people, the neurotoxins inflame the top of the vagus nerve, where it originates in the brain. This is more like vagus nerve–related brain inflammation, and it can account for that chronic boat-like feeling or that experience where the slightest movement or twist of your neck can prompt instant room spins and even vomiting. How serious the dizziness or balance struggle is depends greatly on what kind of condition the liver is in, since the liver is where EBV likes to hide out. Is someone eating foods that could be fueling the virus? How many pesticides and fungicides has someone been exposed to—since these chemicals feed viruses, too?

By the way, Ménière's disease is often blamed on calcium crystals or stones becoming disrupted in the inner ear. This is not accurate. It's a theory that makes the person with dizziness feel like they have an answer when they leave the doctor's office. The truth is that stones have nothing to do with chronic suffering from vertigo, dizziness, the spins, or other balance issues. Ménière's is a real neurological condition caused by chronic, low-grade viral infection.

Celery juice is one of the all-time greatest anti-inflammatories. It is a powerful remedy to stabilize any of these conditions; it addresses all of the concerns around balance struggles. Celery juice components easily drive themselves into the brain, where its trace minerals restore neurons and nourish and replenish nerves, including major central nerves such as the vagus. At the same time, its sodium cluster salts help destroy and kill off EBV. And they do more than that: the cluster salts bind onto neurotoxins, pesticides, herbicides, fungicides, and other poisons inside the liver and the rest of the body and help flush them out to reduce reactions with the vagus nerve. If neurotoxins are sitting on the surface of the vagus nerve, causing it to react, celery juice can magnetically attract the neurotoxins and pull them off the nerve. Essentially what celery juice does is clean up the vagus nerve, dusting off pollutants, toxins, and neurotoxins of any kind, especially the ones from EBV.

BLOATING

Celery juice helps alleviate bloating for a number of reasons. First, it revives the liver, which allows for increased bile production and reserves. More bile production means stronger breakdown and digestion of fats, whether healthy or unhealthy, from the high-fat diets most everyone eats. This bile strength disperses new fats that are being consumed on an ongoing basis as well as old fats that have hardened and caked along the walls of the gut, causing illnesses and symptoms such as bloating.

As celery juice is revitalizing the liver, it's also revitalizing the stomach glands. We rely on these glands to produce an array of gastric juices, some critical to our digestion, processing, and breakdown of nutrients such as proteins. When protein is not being digested properly and is instead rotting in the gut, bloating can occur. Actually, that alone is a cause of chronic bloating for many. Celery juice's sodium cluster salts enter the stomach glands and feed cells there, purging them of any toxins from toxic food chemicals such as preservatives and "natural flavors" (which are MSG-laden—read more in *Medical Medium*). When the stomach gland tissue is revived, the glands can produce stronger hydrochloric acid—which is actually composed of seven different acids—at a higher rate. In turn, this helps break down protein.

Celery juice also kills off SIBO-related pathogens such as strep. (And if you read *Liver Rescue*, then you know medical research and science have yet to discover that strep is the leading type of bacteria in SIBO.) Colonies of unproductive bacteria like strep off-gas ammonia as they feed off undigested proteins and fats in our guts. That ammonia then seeps up the digestive tract, wreaking havoc as it goes, all the way up to the stomach and even mouth, where it can cause receding gums and quicken tooth decay. As celery juice kills off strep and other pathogens while its digestive enzymes help process food in the intestinal tract, it leads to less bloating.

Someone can experience one of these causes of bloating—low bile, low hydrochloric acid, or pathogens off-gassing ammonia—two of them, or all three at once. Most people have more than one, and no matter which cause, the chronic bloating is usually an early sign of a liver condition developing. That's all the more reason to turn to celery juice, since it's such a support for the liver.

BRAIN FOG

Brain fog has two main causes, sometimes occurring separately and sometimes at the same time. One of the leading reasons for brain fog is low-grade viral infection such as the common Epstein-Barr virus residing inside the liver. When EBV fuels itself on troublemakers from our everyday environment that end up in our livers—we're talking old pharmaceuticals; mercury, aluminum, copper, and other toxic heavy metals; solvents; and petrochemicals—it releases neurotoxins that can float around the bloodstream, enter the brain, and dampen or short-circuit electrical impulses there while weakening neurotransmitter chemicals. The result is brain fog. Medical research and science are completely unaware of this cause.

Note that people with viral brain fog don't normally have a virus in the brain itself. Instead they're dealing with a viral infection in the liver. Celery juice's chemical compounds enter the liver via the hepatic portal vein. From there, celery juice's sodium cluster salts attach to viral neurotoxins, disarming them while also disarming EBV's viral cells before they can even reach the brain and cause brain fog.

The other reason someone may experience brain fog is due to toxic heavy metals themselves in the brain. Mercury and aluminum are two of the most common ones that sit in the brain and impede electrical impulses. Electrical impulses tend to short out after running into deposits of toxic heavy metals, resulting in trouble forming clear thoughts. Brain fog is more complicated than people think. There are

hundreds and hundreds of variations, with each person experiencing their own version that's a little different in nature. One reason why brain fog is so different for every single individual is that heavy metal deposits are in different places in the brain for everyone—for some people they're "sprinkled" throughout, while for others, they're more localized. Further, people's brains harbor different varieties, combinations, and levels of heavy metals.

Celery juice's sodium cluster salts help strengthen neurotransmitter chemicals as well as electrical impulses so they have stronger travel velocities and can cover longer distances. With the right fuel, the fire behind the electricity in the brain burns brighter, allowing for greater clarity as it burns though brain fog—and that "right fuel" is precisely what celery juice's sodium cluster salts provide. These sodium cluster salts also detoxify, dislodge, and uproot heavy metals from the brain.

Another result of heavy metals in the brain—and another contributor to brain fog—is oxidation. When toxic heavy metals oxidize, whether because the metals are aging or because there's too much fat in the diet and bloodstream, the heavy metals create runoff that can further interfere with brain function. Celery juice tends to disarm, neutralize, and disperse oxidative material, making more room in and on neurons and brain tissue, giving brain cells freedom from heavy metal contamination. As a result, electrical impulses and neurons can more freely do their jobs, helping alleviate brain fog.

BRITTLE, RIDGED NAILS AND NAIL FUNGUS

Celery juice strengthens damaged, weak, brittle, or ridged nails by restoring the liver. That's right: flushing poisons and toxins from the liver makes for better nails. The reason is that zinc is a treasured mineral in the body. The liver takes whatever precious zinc it can find from any food consumed and converts it into a usable mineral source of healing. If the liver is in good working condition, not sluggish or stagnant, it can release this renewed zinc into the bloodstream to help recover nail issues. When nails are problematic, it's a sign that the liver is problematic and low in zinc. Celery juice contains the mineral zinc in bioavailable form, which can greatly improve nails.

When it's a nail fungus that's the problem, celery juice can help, too, over time. The sodium cluster salts break down and destroy bodily fungus that's not useful. In severe cases, you'll need to take further measures. Combine celery juice with other healing tools, and then you've got truly dramatic healing power. Turn to Chapter 8, "More Healing Guidance," for assistance.

CANCER

Almost all cancers are caused by viruses. The very few cancers that are not viral are caused by toxic chemical agents or industrial chemicals all on their own. Asbestos is one example of a toxin creating cancer without a virus present. The majority of cancers have a viral component. Specifically, they're caused by viruses feeding on toxins. Not that every time you have a virus and toxins present in your body, cancer will form. It takes particular mutated strains of certain viruses to create cancer, and they won't go cancerous unless they have strong enough toxic fuel.

When particular aggressive strains of viruses feed on particular aggressive toxins, the viruses release toxic waste matter that is essentially that original toxin in a more poisonous form. The release of this waste matter poisons healthy cells over and over again. The healthy human cells then die off and provide more fuel for the virus. This cycle continues until cells mutate and turn into cancer cells—while the virus is also mutating to the point that its cells, too, can become cancer cells. This process can occur anywhere in the body, because viruses can travel anywhere in the body. So can toxins.

Celery juice is one of the most profound, preventative anti-cancer herbs or foods. As healthy as munching on a few sticks of celery a day can be, this is not the medicine that celery juice is. Celery juice in the recommended quantities you'll find in the next chapter can do two things for someone who's trying to prevent or cope with cancer. First, it can help remove the toxins that provide fuel for viruses. A few examples of these toxins are foreign hormones that enter from outside the body, toxic heavy metals, toxic medications, and toxic plastics and other petroleum products. Celery juice can bind onto, loosen, and help cast away these toxins from the liver and anywhere else in the body, lowering your toxic load and bettering your chances of preventing cancer. If you're already struggling with cancer, celery juice offers the opportunity to slow it down and prevent future cancers by removing these same toxins and poisons. Second, celery juice is an antiviral. Its sodium cluster salts help destroy the aggressive viruses that like to consume toxins and excrete more-poisonous toxins—the process that denatures and damages cells to the point that they eventually become cancerous. By taking away viruses' power, celery juice helps interrupt cancer from forming or spreading. So it's a win on both sides: celery juice addresses toxins *and* viruses.

The vitamin C in celery juice is a powerful antioxidant that assimilates very easily and feeds cancer-killing cells inside the body. Celery juice's plant hormones restore the endocrine system, keeping it from becoming overactive—which is helpful because a lot of fight-or-flight in the body can release a lot of fear-based adrenaline, another fuel for viral cancer cells.

Most people suffering from cancer are already working with compassionate, highly trained physicians and receiving natural treatments, conventional treatments, or both. Talk to your doctor about adding celery juice to whatever cancer protocol you're already following. If you're a cancer survivor, celery juice is a fantastic preventative for relapses, because it can gather up toxins and poisons that could be accumulating as fuel for viruses, and then it can send them out of the body.

CHILLS, HOT FLASHES, NIGHT SWEATS, RUNNING HOT, AND TEMPERATURE FLUCTUATIONS

These symptoms are all connected to a sluggish, stagnant liver filled with a variety of toxins—including toxic hormones from years of fight-or-flight; toxic heavy metals such as mercury, aluminum, and copper; poisonous viral waste matter from viruses such as Epstein-Barr, HHV-6, shingles, and even cytomegalovirus; along with pharmaceuticals and exposure to pesticides, herbicides, and fungicides. When the liver is burdened with all this at the same time it's working hard to defend itself against a high-fat diet—which almost everyone is on, regardless of whether it's regarded as "healthy"—the liver eventually maxes out. This happens for different people at different times in life. Some people are born with a sluggish, stagnant liver from toxins passed on from earlier generations, so these symptoms can arise earlier. For many, these symptoms come in the late 30s, early 40s, or 50s.

Celery juice is a tonic for all of this. It enters the liver through the hepatic portal vein and then sets about reviving and revitalizing damaged liver cells, loosening and removing debris and toxic troublemakers, neutralizing viral waste such as neurotoxins and dermatoxins, and breaking down and dispersing fat cells. This ultimately results in fresher, cleaner blood, so that when the bloodstream directs it to enter the liver again, it's less toxic. Essentially, celery juice brings the liver back to life, lowering the toxic load that most everyone develops as they go through life. With a renewed and refreshed liver, these temperature-related symptoms can improve. This is a case where supplementing celery juice with an improved diet really helps—see Chapter 8, "More Healing Guidance."

COLD HANDS AND FEET; SENSITIVITY TO COLD, HEAT, SUN EXPOSURE, OR HUMIDITY

People who struggle with temperature sensitivities are normally dealing with a sensitive nervous system. Nerves and nerve endings in various parts of the body, from the trigeminal nerve to other facial nerves to the sciatic nerve, become sensitive because they are inflamed. Celery juice goes to the source of that inflammation.

Those who can handle extreme cold or extreme heat don't know what it's like to experience a 50-degree day as nearly painful. Wind, too, can feel biting to someone with sensitive facial nerves. People with these sensitivities often get headaches or migraines easily or feel their sense of balance affected, becoming dizzy or even developing mild vertigo periodically. Cold weather can wipe them out, or hot weather can make them feel just as bad. Some people are very sensitive to standing in the sun too long, or they can't cope with heavy humidity. No matter what name you put on someone's experience or what condition

a doctor diagnoses this as, it's happening because of a sensitive nervous system.

When nerve sensitivities are not due to physical injury, nerves are inflamed due to an elevated viral load in the body. Viruses such as Epstein-Barr are responsible for so many different neurological conditions and symptoms. These viruses release their form of waste matter called neurotoxins, which float through the bloodstream, attaching themselves to nerves and causing the nerves to become anywhere from slightly to extremely inflamed, depending on the person and the viral load. That's what leads to a heightened reaction to temperature. When someone is experiencing cold extremities, it's due to these viral neurotoxins plus circulation issues from a sluggish liver.

Celery juice's unique sodium cluster salts are so grounding that they get to work right away neutralizing and binding onto neurotoxins, rendering them less aggressive and helping them leave the body more quickly through urination, elimination, or even perspiration. This allows nerves to relax and heal, which lowers nerve inflammation throughout the body. Then, when the body naturally swells in a time of high humidity, there isn't as much pressure on the nerves, so someone doesn't have to suffer. Fewer neurotoxins impeding nerves throughout the body also means that when someone is exposed to cold, the nerves bounce back more quickly, resulting in less pain and exhaustion.

CONSTANT HUNGER

A result of glucose deficiency inside your organs, constant hunger is a sign in particular of a hungry liver, one that's starving for new glycogen (stored glucose) deposits. Oftentimes, the liver is congested with built-up fat cells from high-fat diets as well as toxins and other troublemakers. This makes it harder for the liver to receive glucose, which is why it's possible to consistently eat a lot and still feel hungry. Celery juice helps flush these toxins out of the liver and dissolve and disperse fat cells, opening the door for glucose absorption and glycogen storage, which you can get from fresh fruits, potatoes, and other starchy vegetables such as winter squash. Learn more about these *critical clean carbohydrates* (CCC) in Chapter 8 of this book and in *Liver Rescue*.

CONSTIPATION

The digestive enzymes alone in celery juice can help break down food in the small intestinal tract and get your system moving when you're having an off day and feeling backed up. Celery juice is also there to assist when constipation is more of a chronic problem.

Most people who are dealing with constipation are dealing with a sluggish, stagnant liver. When this happens with younger folks, it could be because you came into this life with a liver burdened with toxins passed down from your ancestors. If you're older, a sluggish liver could have been building for

decades. Maybe you, too, started life with a compromised liver, and then a lifetime of eating the type of high-fat diet we're conditioned to consume put the liver on overload. An overburdened, weakened liver results in lower bile production, and bile is critical for digesting the fats in our diets. When bile diminishes, fats don't break down or disperse as they should, and they end up going rancid in our guts, feeding colonies of unproductive bacteria.

Another way digestion can get interrupted is when hydrochloric acid weakens in the stomach. (Find out more about the complex seven-acid blend that your stomach produces in *Liver Rescue*.) If the stomach glands are forced to overproduce hydrochloric acid over the years to compensate for a damaged or weakened liver, they'll eventually lose strength, and the resulting lower levels of gastric juices mean that proteins will not break down properly, regardless of whether those are plant- or animal-based proteins. Those proteins will rot in the gut and, again, feed colonies of unproductive bacteria.

When unproductive bacteria proliferate in the digestive tract, inflammation occurs and peristaltic action starts to minimize. "Hot spots" can develop in the small intestinal tract and colon; that is, places where pockets of bacteria develop or a narrowing occurs, causing more constipation over time. So many people with constipation these days get diagnosed with small intestinal bacterial overgrowth (SIBO), especially in the alternative medicine world. Medical research and science are unaware that the leading type of bacteria in SIBO is *Strepto-coccus* and that there are dozens of strep varieties that are not yet identified.

The sodium cluster salts in celery juice are the ultimate pathogen destroyers. They immediately start destroying colonies of unproductive bacteria, including strep, making celery juice a critical remedy for constipation (and SIBO). Unlike how strep can become resistant to antibiotics, strep can't become immune to the cluster salts in celery juice. They keep working. As you read in the previous chapter, this in turn keeps feeding beneficial bacteria in the gut.

Celery juice also revitalizes a sluggish, stagnant liver so that bile production is replenished. It revives the stomach glands, too, so that hydrochloric acid production can be restored: the stomach glands that produce hydrochloric acid find trace minerals specifically in celery juice that feed their tissue.

Sometimes constipation is a result of kinks in the small intestinal tract or colon. These are not obstructions; rather, weakened connective tissue around the intestines can create a gentle kinking that makes it difficult for somebody to have a bowel movement. Often this is also the result of a toxic liver—the connective tissue around the intestines has weakened because it's become saturated with toxins, bacteria, and viruses that the liver has become too overburdened to filter. These troublemakers also end up inside the intestinal tract. Food choice can contribute, too. Some people need more peristalsis-related food if they aren't getting enough fiber. An easy

remedy for many is adding a little more plant-based food to the diet overall. Celery juice is also an amazing peristaltic contributor. (That's true even though it doesn't have fiber—to help clear up any confusion over fiber, see "The Fiber Question" in Chapter 4 and also visit Chapter 7, "Rumors, Concerns, and Myths.") Celery juice naturally triggers peristaltic action; if someone's not getting enough fiber in their everyday diet, celery juice can stimulate peristalsis to move food along through the intestines. Further, celery juice can help with kinks in the small intestinal tract and colon by reestablishing the intestines' inner linings and rejuvenating connective tissue around them.

And then there's emotional constipation. Holding in too long or going through emotional struggles, worries, stress, hardships, and betrayals can create internal tension and unrest that leads to constipation. In these situations, celery juice helps the brain greatly. Its intense electrolyte power reestablishes neurotransmitter chemicals, essentially relaxing and cooling down the mind and brain. When its sodium cluster salts enter into neurons and feed them, it can alter someone's state of being, ultimately leading to peristaltic action.

DIABETES (TYPES 1, 1.5, AND 2), HYPERGLYCEMIA, AND HYPOGLYCEMIA

Early insulin resistance symptoms such as hypoglycemia, hyperglycemia, or an elevated A1C start from a sluggish, stagnant liver. When the liver weakens, its ability to digest fats diminishes, leading to larger volumes of fat buildup in the gut, around other organs, and even in the bloodstream. This is what leads to insulin resistance. Plus, when the liver accumulates fat, it loses its strength to control and store glucose in the form of precious glycogen reserves. Celery juice revives the liver, allowing it to dissolve and purge built-up fat that it stored away to protect the brain and heart from an overload of fat. As it returns to vitality, a healthy liver can preserve and release glycogen reserves as needed to prevent insulin resistance.

Reviving the liver is how celery juice helps with type 2 diabetes as well. Along with the proper dietary recommendations, which you'll find throughout the Medical Medium series, celery juice is very helpful for healing type 2 diabetes. Once the liver springs back to life thanks to celery juice and other dietary support—its liver lobules are revitalized, old fats are cleansed from the liver, and glucose storage is working properly once more—the pancreas can begin to rejuvenate more quickly. Stronger bile reserves can build up, too, so that bile can break down and disperse fats more robustly. Less fat hanging around in the bloodstream means that when any kind of carbohydrate, whether healthy or unhealthy, enters the body, the insulin resistance that so often leads to type 2 diabetes doesn't occur as easily.

Types 1 and 1.5 diabetes (the second of which is also known as latent autoimmune diabetes in adults, or LADA) are caused by pancreas damage, whether from pathogenic

activity or physical injury. Viruses can enter into the pancreas, attacking it and causing pancreatic inflammation, which can lead to a chronic diabetic condition. Theorists claim that types 1 and 1.5 diabetes are autoimmune; that is, that the body's own immune system is attacking the pancreas. Don't get caught up in this confusion. In cases where a physical blow to the pancreas is not the cause, the truth is that an invading pathogen is what's going after the pancreas, and the immune system is reacting to try to save the gland. These pathogens are highly allergic to celery juice's sodium cluster salts; when celery juice enters the system, it helps kill them off. And remember, the plant hormones in celery juice help stabilize and strengthen all the endocrine glands in the body, including the pancreas. This means that long-term use of celery juice can help improve someone's type 1 or 1.5 diabetes, provided they also become aware of better dietary guidelines such as lowering fat intake as well as proper supplementation to reduce any kind of viral load inside the pancreas. As insulin resistance lowers, less supplemental insulin is needed.

People sometimes ask if celery juice is safe for diabetics in the first place. As you've just seen, the answer is yes. Celery juice is a godsend for diabetics. What isn't good for diabetics is including foods such as eggs, cheese, pork, milk, and butter in the diet. For a more in-depth understanding of why that is, and fuller explanations of the different varieties of diabetes, turn to *Liver Rescue* and *Medical Medium*.

DIARRHEA

The rumor is that celery juice *causes* diarrhea. Ultimately, it helps alleviate diarrhea. When someone gets the runs after drinking celery juice, it is a temporary healing reaction: an indication that the gut is filled with unproductive bacteria (such as strep), funguses, maybe some viruses, pockets of mucus, and a little bit of mold and yeast. The liver, too, could be full of sludge from bugs and troublemakers: anything from detergents to conventional cleaners to cosmetics, perfumes, and colognes to toxic heavy metals such as mercury, aluminum, and copper to petrochemicals such as gasoline to pesticides, fungicides, and herbicides. Some people already have irritable bowel syndrome (IBS), meaning that the intestinal tract, gallbladder, and liver could already be inflamed. When there's so much toxicity and inflammation going on, dropping celery juice in there means that its sodium cluster salts are hitting everything—killing bugs, flushing out the liver—and diarrhea can result because there's already an underlying condition. Cluster salts are cleaning agents. Depending on how toxic someone's system is, the healing reaction can vary. Some people's systems are more overloaded with pathogens and other troublemakers. When that's the case, it can make sense to start with less than 16 ounces and work up from there.

When someone is experiencing diarrhea without drinking celery juice, it could have many different causes. A common one is a negative reaction to foods such as eggs; dairy products, including milk, cheese, and butter; gluten; and even soy and corn. These foods feed pathogens residing in the gut, from the stomach all the way down to the colon and rectum. Strep is a very common bug that loves to feast on these foods. So do EBV, shingles, and aggressive, unfriendly varieties of fungus (not including *Candida*, which is friendly). Proliferation of these bugs can lead to an imbalance in the gut, with not enough productive microorganisms present to keep the unproductive ones in check. As a result, the unhelpful bugs multiply, which can lead somebody to become chronically inflamed all through the small intestine and colon. Pockets can expand in the intestinal tract, and some areas can even shrink, leading to diagnoses of Crohn's disease, celiac disease, SIBO, IBS, and even colitis. Symptoms can range from mild bowel irritation to severe ulcers and inflammation to somebody just living life with a little bit of diarrhea that never gets diagnosed.

Celery juice helps reverse diarrhea by destroying and eliminating these unproductive varieties of bacteria and viruses. It weakens them, breaks them down, and helps flush them out of the digestive tract. Celery juice also helps feed productive bacteria with trace minerals and special protective, strengthening antioxidants that only celery juice possesses so that these beneficial microorganisms can reestablish themselves at healthy levels. Once the pathogen load reduces, the liver starts to revitalize and flush out poisons, the intestinal tract pushes out toxins, and chronic inflammation drops dramatically, freeing somebody of diarrhea.

If inflammation had reached beyond the gut all the way to the pancreas, celery juice helps rid the pathogens that caused this and revive pancreatic tissue as well. People who consume celery juice long term can rid themselves of diarrhea completely, especially if they're following dietary and supplemental guidance from the rest of the Medical Medium series. Start with Chapter 8 for ideas.

DRY, CRACKED SKIN

Dry skin is one of the first indications of dehydration. Chronically dry, cracked skin often happens when the blood is filled with a combination of fats and toxins. Fats block oxygen from easily entering the dermis, and oxygen is critical for healthy skin. Most everyone has a large amount of fat in their diet, and even healthy fats thicken up the blood and minimize oxygen, allowing toxins to fester. These toxins can saturate the tissue below the skin and push up under the dermis, causing the skin to crack as it tries to release them. A sluggish, fatty liver filled with toxins is a recipe for dry, cracked skin because that's what results in the dirtier, less oxygenated blood that causes this situation.

Celery juice assists by cleaning up the liver, binding onto toxins, disarming and neutralizing them, and flushing them out of the body. It also binds onto and disperses fats in the bloodstream, allowing fats to leave the body more easily. There's no quick way to remedy dry, cracked skin, because a sluggish, stagnant liver filled with viral debris, toxic heavy metals, and other toxins takes some time to remedy. On its own, the liver cleanses so many toxins on a daily basis. If someone's liver is very toxic—and the majority of people's are—then the liver's mere act of doing its daily job is impeded, and it struggles. This alone allows ample amounts of toxins to surface and saturate the dermis because the liver can't hold on to them, so they enter the bloodstream and from there, reach the skin. Because the liver is too burdened, it doesn't get a chance to disarm and neutralize the troublemakers, so when they reach the dermis, they're more aggressive.

Once you put the liver in a cleanse state (whether through a good, healthy, safe cleanse such as the Celery Juice Cleanse from Chapter 5 or an unproductive cleanse like the countless ones out there), it starts to flush out toxins. During that time, you're still going to experience dry, cracked skin for a while, because some toxins are going to enter the dermis and exit through the skin. Long-term diligence and dedication with celery juice and other Medical Medium techniques, such as those you'll find in *Liver Rescue*, can clean enough toxins out of the liver and bloodstream to finally reverse dry, cracked skin.

EATING DISORDERS

There are different varieties of eating disorders and different causes. Recognizable eating disorders are usually in the realm of anorexia, bulimia, and overeating. These can be caused by emotional distress, afflictions, or extreme stress; toxic heavy metal exposure; societal expectations of how we're supposed to look; or some combination of all of these. Chronic illness can also cause digestive compromises and confusion about what to eat and when to eat, and this can lead to eating disorders. Then there are the eating disorders that go unidentified—because the truth is that every person on the planet has an eating disorder of some kind. It may not be extreme. It may not be obvious. It's still there, whether stemming from childhood difficulties or toxic exposure, creating hang-ups or unproductive patterns around food.

Celery juice can help with all of these. For one, it helps restore neurotransmitter chemicals: sodium cluster salts and the trace minerals connected to them provide the ultimate neurotransmitter chemicals for the brain. For another, celery juice makes neurons stronger and electricity in the brain more dynamic and free, allowing for emotional wounds to heal faster. When electrical impulses aren't intercepted or impeded by deposits of toxic heavy metals such as mercury and aluminum—the cause of so many eating disorders—healthy thought patterns can establish themselves. Celery juice's status as the ultimate electrolyte source for the brain can prompt healing for so many other causes of eating disorders, too.

Not to mention that the plant hormones in celery juice help restore the entire endocrine system. People with eating disorders tend to have compromised endocrine glands—particularly the adrenals—and plant hormones provide vital chemical compounds to help restore them. Plant hormones help brain cells communicate with each other, too, further allowing people to overcome emotional aspects of eating disorders.

Celery juice also rebuilds hydrochloric acid in the stomach, which helps people who are suffering from bulimia recover. It aids in reducing inflammation of the intestinal tract as well by killing off pathogens such as unproductive bacteria that reside there. This brings someone back to health after dealing with digestive issues that interfered with eating, so they don't have to live in fear and confusion around food anymore.

EDEMA AND SWELLING

Swollen or Puffy Eyes, Face, Neck, Hands, Upper Arms, Feet, Ankles, Calves, Thighs, or Abdomen

If someone is struggling with puffiness, swelling, or edema and hasn't been diagnosed with a heart condition, kidney disease, or other condition that directly explains it, then it is a mystery to medical research and science. Millions of people walk around with all types of edema and no explanation from their physician about what's causing it. Doctors know that sometimes edema is a side effect of pharmaceuticals, although they don't realize that even when edema is not a known, direct side effect, a drug can still result in swelling if it's bogging down or weakening the liver.

Most variations of edema that aren't heart- or kidney-related are related to the liver, whether a pharmaceutical is involved or not.

What's happening inside the liver to cause it? This is yet another outcome of a stagnant, sluggish liver filled with toxins. In this case, there will most often be a viral infection of the liver, too, going unnoticed and undiagnosed by a physician. Often, people experiencing edema or puffiness are experiencing other symptoms, too, and nobody realizes it all traces back to this same undiscovered viral infection. People with Hashimoto's, fibromyalgia, ME/CFS, Lyme disease, RA, or MS, for example, will also experience mild to severe edema, and a viral infection inside the liver is what started all of it. Sometimes more than one virus is in play, including different strains and mutations of Epstein-Barr and shingles. Strep, too, can proliferate in the liver, and both viruses and bacteria can create a tremendous amount of byproduct and debris. One of your body's defense mechanisms when large deposits of toxic sludge like this build up in your liver is to send it to your lymphatic system. As a result, your lymphatic system swells, collecting water trying to dilute the toxins. The lymphatic system is not designed to handle an abundance of viral and bacterial byproduct and debris. It's designed for normal, everyday environmental pollutants, toxins that our body produces, and toxins that we encounter from food. Our lymphatic system was never meant to be pathogens' punching bag, taking blows from large amounts of viral and bacterial waste matter while also handling its main responsibility, an influx of troublemakers from daily life.

Celery juice helps flush these waste deposits from the lymphatic system. It also helps break down and destroy pathogens inside the liver, which lowers the viral load while also helping reduce the toxic load in the liver (and other organs), flushing it into the bloodstream and continuing to carry it out of the body. All of this reduces water retention.

By the way, the water of water retention isn't pretty. When we experience swelling and fluid buildup, it's not clean and clear fluid; it's discolored, usually carrying a yellow, mucus-y tinge. It's also usually thicker and mucus-like in consistency, too, because it's dirty, filled with toxins and viral waste. Celery juice helps clear up that viscous, tinted water, cleaning it and renewing it, since sodium cluster salts have the unique ability to neutralize toxins and purify fluids inside of our body, allowing fluids to flow through the body and release trapped toxins with ease.

EMOTIONAL STRUGGLES

Anxiousness, Anxiety, Mood Swings, Guilt, Sadness, Irritability, Bipolar Disorder, and Depression

Nobody wants to be irritable or down or worried or chronically guilty or experience frequent mood swings. Everybody wants to live their life feeling good, happy, clear, and at peace. When we're talking about mental health, we always need to start with this knowledge. Far too often we tell people struggling with their emotions that it's all a matter of mind-set and that they just need to shift their perspective. When it's women who are dealing with emotional challenges, far too often they hear that it's hormones, too. That's a sign that medical research and science don't have a full handle on mental health.

Celery juice helps bring the goodness, happiness, clarity, and peace we're all seeking because it directly addresses the true cause behind mood struggles: toxins. Now, difficult life events and circumstances can create some irritability, anxiousness, and sadness on their own. Understanding cause and effect there is usually clear. Celery juice can help then, because it rejuvenates brain tissue, including in the emotional centers of the brain, where we can sustain emotional injuries. When we're talking about chronic emotional troubles that surface when life seems to be going along at its normal pace, with no discernible triggering event, that's when we're talking about toxins. Everyone has a unique brew of toxins inside their body. The toxic load that some people carry is more disruptive to neurotransmitters and neurons inside the brain, and that's part of what accounts for the variability in mental health.

One thing that most people have in common is a toxic buildup of heavy metals, viral toxins, or both, usually inside the liver. What do I mean by "viral toxins"? When certain viruses—which love to hide out in the liver—consume their favorite foods, such as toxic heavy metals, eggs, and synthetic

chemicals that they find there in the liver, they tend to release neurotoxins. (This is too bad, since so many people are told that eating eggs is healthy.) These neurotoxins then float around the body and can find their way to the brain, where they hinder neurotransmitter chemicals and weaken electrical impulses throughout the brain. This can cause irritability, anxiousness, anxiety, mood swings, and even fluctuations in behavior and mood that could be diagnosed as bipolar. The severity of the symptom will often vary with the severity of the toxic heavy metals and the degree of the viral load, and what type of viral mutation is residing in the liver.

A common virus that releases these neurotoxins is Epstein-Barr, and there are over 60 strains of EBV alone. Different viral strains have different appetites for different foods. And again, since everyone has a different toxic brew—different toxic heavy metals as well as different pesticides, herbicides, and other substances—add that to the viral variability and it accounts for the varying degrees of anxiousness, depression, and more that people can experience. Some people have a higher viral load in the liver, where a virus is gobbling down its favorite pesticides, herbicides, gluten, eggs, and dairy products and releasing an abundance of neurotoxins that make their way to the brain through the bloodstream, resulting in milder forms of depression, bipolar behavior, and anxiety.

Everyone is their own unique soul and individual, and no one's levels of viral toxins or heavy metals will be the same. This means that how each person experiences their emotional struggles is going to be entirely unique. How neurotoxins end up saturating the brain, diminishing or weakening neurotransmitter chemicals, and impeding electrical activity is going to affect one person one way, another person another way, and so on and so on and so on. The same goes for toxic heavy metals that end up inside the brain. How mercury, aluminum, copper, or other heavy metals land and in what quantity will affect how they ignite bouts of depression, bipolar behavior, looming sadness, or unexplained guilt and what those feel like to someone. From person to person, these emotional states could feel completely different. In the case of more pronounced bipolar disorder and depression, there are often more toxic heavy metals residing in the brain itself, short-circuiting electrical impulses and neurotransmitters. General moodiness usually results from an all-around overload of toxins in the body, both a cause and a result of a stagnant, sluggish liver. Emotional wounds can combine with toxic heavy metals or a viral load inside the liver to create more pronounced irritability, anxiousness, or full-blown anxiety.

Celery juice has different timing for helping alleviate emotional struggles for each person. Someone with irritability could improve after one week of drinking celery juice daily. Someone with severe anxiety or depression or any other pronounced emotional struggle could take longer, although the condition can start getting more livable and bearable early on and keep getting better and better.

Drinking celery juice is like allowing a breath of fresh air to enter your consciousness. It's a cleaning agent that enters the brain, rounding up and flushing toxins to free up brain tissue that's been saturated for years and years by neurotoxin and toxic heavy metal buildup. Celery juice's power in restoring mental health comes from its sodium cluster salts, which revitalize and provide neurotransmitter chemicals, cleaning and renewing tattered ones and also offering complete neurotransmitter chemicals so that neurons can function as they're meant to inside the brain. These cluster salts also gather toxins inside the brain—including toxic heavy metals such as mercury, aluminum, and copper—helping to disarm, neutralize, and disperse them. They remove neurotoxins from neurotransmitters and neurons by binding onto them and forcing them to disperse while revitalizing brain cells at the same time.

Most everyone's brain is undernourished from poor diet (because we're not taught what truly healthy diets are), an overabundance of stress, and toxic exposure. Over time, this exhausts our brains. Celery juice is like a multivitamin for the brain—one of the best overall brain cell rejuvenators and enhancers. Cell by cell, celery juice reestablishes your brain's health so that it can heal naturally on its own. At the same time, celery juice addresses the specific troublemakers that interfere with our emotions.

Celery juice's sodium cluster salts also lower the pathogen levels responsible for neurotoxins in the first place. They strip away and break down viruses' outer cell membranes, weakening them to allow your immune system to destroy the pathogens. Further, celery juice cleans up the liver and even supports the adrenal glands. Trace mineral salts are the ultimate fuel for the adrenals—and anyone with anxiousness, anxiety, mood swings, guilt, sadness, irritability, bipolar disorder, or depression is dealing with adrenal complications, whether adrenal weakness or even adrenal fatigue. That's because the uneasy feelings that accompany these conditions put the adrenals on constant fight-or-flight alert. It's very difficult to deal with fatigue on top of emotional struggles. When celery juice revitalizes and strengthens the adrenals, it allows you to have more energy, which is a key part of recovery.

EYE PROBLEMS

When we think about eating for eye health, we often think about vitamin A and orange and red pigments—beta-carotene and carotenoids—as being helpful for the eyes. What's even better are antioxidants from foods such as berries: the blues in wild blueberries, for example, and the deep colors of raspberries and blackberries. It would be hard to believe, then, that celery juice can do even better than these rich pigments. And yet it can.

Eye health is compromised by toxins that medical research and science aren't aware are interfering. Toxic heavy metals are some of the most antagonistic troublemakers for the eyes. Traces of mercury can easily enter into someone's eye from metal amalgam dental fillings alone. (Although be careful about getting metal fillings removed. That can release mercury, too—read more in *Medical Medium*.) There's also mercury in our water, mercury in our fish, and we're exposed to mercury from generations before us, because we inherit it through our family blood line. That's how the majority of mercury enters into our eyes—passed down from our ancestors through sperm and egg (and also in utero) for generation after generation. It's not the disease itself coming from family members; it's this heavy metal. Degenerative eye diseases of all kinds have mercury involved, even if medical research and science are decades from realizing this. Heavy metals are behind mysterious blindness that's considered genetic; cells inside our eyes that are responsible for vision get saturated with corrosive aluminum byproduct that's a result of interactions with mercury.

Another annoying nuisance factor for eye health is viral activity. Someone can have herpes simplex activity for years, and it can eventually affect the eyes. Simplex 1, shingles varieties, many different EBV varieties, cytomegalovirus, and HHV-6 are all candidates for producing antagonistic toxins and byproduct that slowly degrade the retina or other parts of the eye.

Celery juice is one of the most powerful foods for vision and restoration of the eyes. In this area, it equals and even surpasses the wild blueberry, which is the only other food on Planet Earth that has the power to protect your eyes to this degree. Wild blueberries help the eyes because of their antioxidants. With celery juice, one reason why it's healing people is that it helps remove toxic copper from the body. Sodium cluster salts contain trace minerals that are critical for the eyes, including trace zinc and trace copper. The trace mineral zinc shuts down any kind of viral activity around and inside the eye, even along the optic nerve, while the trace mineral copper binds onto toxic copper and helps loosen and dislodge it so it floats out of the eye, into the bloodstream, and eventually out of the body. The trace zinc also helps interrupt reactions of mercury and aluminum that lead to corrosion and degenerative eye disease.

Vitamin C from celery juice enters the eye hitched on to the sodium cluster salts. While the cluster salts help renew and restore eye tissue, vitamin C can enter cells with them. Almost anyone with any eye problem of any kind has a deficiency in vitamin C because almost anyone with an eye problem has a liver problem. A liver that's sluggish, stagnant, overburdened, or dysfunctional means that it's unable to customize the vitamin C that enters it—unable to methylate it properly to make it more bioavailable and accessible for the rest of the body. Celery juice's vitamin C provides an instant infusion for the eye cells, sustaining them and helping them reverse or at least halt the advance of disease. Neurons in the brain that send signals to the optic nerve also rely on celery juice's sodium cluster

salts because of the improvement to neurotransmitters that they bring. This alone can assist with a multitude of eye symptoms, from basic to extreme.

Now let's take a look at how celery juice helps several specific eye symptoms and conditions. Even if you don't see your particular issue in this list, rest assured, celery juice is there for you.

Cataracts

The cause here is a long-term vitamin C deficiency from an overburdened, toxic liver that's loaded down with pesticides, herbicides, fungicides, and old DDT. Celery juice helps prevent growth of cataracts by unburdening the liver while providing potent, usable vitamin C.

Color Blindness

Exposure to aluminum toxicity deep within and throughout the eye in utero or shortly after birth is what results in color blindness. People who are color blind also tend to experience eye sensitivities as they age because of this aluminum exposure. Celery juice helps prevent and address these additional sensitivities and conditions.

Congenital Eye Defects

These issues are considered to be passed through genes. Medical research and science are unaware that what's really being passed on from generations before are toxic heavy metals, which tend to build up from generation to generation. Mercury is the leading toxic heavy metal to cause eye defects at birth. Celery juice helps protect cells in the eye from further mercury damage as the years pass into adulthood, because it helps prevent mercury from expanding.

Conjunctivitis (Pink Eye)

Conjunctivitis is a chronic bacterial infection caused by *Streptococcus*. There are acute versions of conjunctivitis and long-term, serious ones, and which condition occurs depends on what variety of strep is present and whether it's a stronger, antibiotic-resistant strain. Celery juice provides sodium cluster salts and easily accessible vitamin C to help minimize strep bacterial colonies that reside deep within the eye and around the eye socket in order to fight the infection. Strep bacteria cannot become immune to celery juice's cluster salts.

Corneal Disease

This occurs from chronic, long-term viral infection. Epstein-Barr is the most common virus behind it. The cloudy material involved is the virus discharging byproduct that builds up inside the eye. Celery juice reduces the viral infection because its sodium cluster salts help destroy the virus, protecting eye cells from viral invasion. It also provides vital vitamin C to protect an eye deficient in the nutrient.

Diabetic Retinopathy

When someone with retinopathy also has diabetes, by default they're going to be said to be connected. That's a mistake. Many people have retinopathy without diabetes, too. Anyone with diabetes has the same problem as anyone without diabetes: a sluggish, stagnant, or fatty liver overburdened with a variety of pesticides, herbicides, petrochemicals, solvents, toxic heavy metals, and viruses. Most everyone with retinopathy, diabetic or not, is largely on a high-fat diet. All of the sugary foods we associate with diabetes—cakes, cookies, doughnuts, and more—are as fatty as they are sugary, and it's that fat that creates problems for the liver, whether it results in a diagnosis of diabetes or someone lives with undiagnosed blood sugar issues. A weakened liver means severe nutrient deficiencies throughout the body, since the liver is the storage bin and delivery system for vitamins and other nutrients, and that's what leads to retinopathy. Celery juice cleanses and slowly restores the liver, which can minimize and even reduce retinopathy.

Dry Eye Syndrome

Most cases of dry eye are the result of chronic dehydration. Soft drinks, coffee, and not enough clean, pure water, coconut water, juices, or fresh fruits leave a person dehydrated long term. So can too much cooked food, which provides very little high-quality, vibrant, living water to nourish cells. When the body is chronically dehydrated, dry eyes and skin are some of the first symptoms because the body is more concerned with protecting the brain and heart. Celery juice rehydrates the body, starting with the liver, and this revives the organ, bringing back its living water storage bin that we examined in *Liver Rescue*; minimizing the toxic, dirty blood that most people walk around with every day; and also rehydrating the lymphatic system to provide critical electrolytes throughout the body.

Some cases of dry eye are caused by underactive adrenals. In these cases, celery juice's sodium cluster salts enter into tired adrenals and help replenish them.

Eye Floaters

Celery juice helps with eye floaters by reducing inflammation that occurs on the optic nerve—which is what's responsible for this mystery symptom that confuses medical research and science. White spots, flares, white flashes, or black spots that occur without noticeable damage to the retina, pupil, or any other part of the eye are the result of neurotoxins from the Epstein-Barr virus, combined with heavy metals such as mercury, inflaming the optic nerve. The powerful flavonoids and vitamin C that travel with celery juice's sodium cluster salts aid specific nerves in and around the brain, including the optic nerve. They disperse neurotoxins that have been sitting on the nerve, and they even protect the nerve from viral invasion while feeding nerve cells, allowing the optic nerve to rejuvenate.

Glaucoma

Glaucoma is caused by a variety of EBV invading the eye, creating inflammation that spurs fluids to develop, and this inflammation and fluid combined elevate eye pressure. The sodium cluster salts and viable, accessible vitamin C in celery juice enter the eye, building up the eye's immune cells and helping break down and destroy EBV.

Low Vision

Mysterious vision weakness where the cause can't be diagnosed is the result of nerve cells inside the optic nerve weakening and diminishing due to various toxins, both viral toxins and toxins from sources such as pesticides, herbicides, fungicides, and petrochemicals. With the use of celery juice, the optic nerve can regenerate. With its high electrolyte count, celery juice helps restore optic nerve cells. Trace minerals and sodium cluster salts provide cells with an infusion that allows new nerve cells to regenerate in the optic nerve. This can help stop low vision from worsening and increase someone's ability to recover and experience improvement.

Macular Degeneration

Macular degeneration is caused by a combination of both toxic heavy metals and viral activity. As you've already read, celery juice helps address both of these, getting to the root of the problem.

Optic Nerve Atrophy

In this more advanced version of mysterious low vision, nerve cells weaken due to toxic heavy metals, petrochemicals, solvents, pesticides, herbicides, fungicides, and/or viral neurotoxins saturating the optic nerve. Degeneration of optic nerve cells occurs, which interferes with messages transferred from the eye to the brain. In some cases of optic nerve atrophy, it's solely a viral infection. EBV is the most common viral cause, HHV-6 is the second, and shingles is the third most likely to invade the optic nerve, creating inflammation that can lead to various diagnoses from doctors who don't realize it's viral. Celery juice's sodium cluster salts help remove viruses from the optic nerve at the same time they restore optic nerve cells, also allowing for new cell growth to proliferate. Further, thanks to its replenishment of neurotransmitter chemicals, celery juice strengthens neurons adjacent to the optic nerve, ones that receive information from the nerve. This increased strength of neurons helps greatly with optic nerve atrophy.

FATIGUE

Daily fatigue with no rhyme or reason, such as the fatigue that goes along with ME/CFS, is often caused by a chronic viral load. Commonly, it's the Epstein-Barr virus. When feeding off harmful substances such as the toxic heavy metal mercury, pesticides, herbicides, pharmaceuticals, and petroleum-based products, EBV produces neurotoxins that float around the body, creating nervous system sensitivities and allergic reactions—resulting in what I call *neurological fatigue*. If this is the kind of fatigue someone is battling, celery juice is helpful because of its extremely antiviral nature. Sodium cluster salts travel through the body in search of viral toxins and even active viruses themselves, stripping viral membranes, in turn causing viral cells to slowly diminish and break down. At the same time, the cluster salts disarm free-floating neurotoxins that are saturating brain tissue and hindering or injuring neurons and neurotransmitter chemicals there. They also disarm neurotoxins that are saturating the heart, liver, pancreas, or even the lungs. By neutralizing these toxins on a daily basis with celery juice, people can gain back stamina over time. Combined with other antiviral measures, they can return to the energy levels they were used to having before—or even better.

If someone's fatigue is really and truly only adrenal fatigue from tired-out adrenal glands and they're experiencing symptoms like being tired all day and then coming to life at night, or getting tired partway through the day and needing a small nap to keep going, celery juice provides the ultimate electrolytes and feeds the adrenal glands with sodium cluster salts that allow the adrenal glands to rebuild, rejuvenate, and restore themselves. As the adrenals strengthen, they tend to stabilize instead of cycling through overworking and underworking, and that helps bring someone back from adrenal fatigue. For more on the adrenals, see "Adrenal Complications."

Exercise fatigue is another type that celery juice can address. This is the result of someone overusing muscles and exhausting the nervous system, from whatever type of exercise that may be. Runners and other athletes can identify this feeling as "hitting a wall." Some non-athletes who haven't built up their strength and endurance may experience exercise fatigue after working out on a basic level for 10 minutes. Either way, celery juice is a miracle worker, reviving muscles better than anything else can. It also helps support nerves inside the muscles, feeding both the nerves and muscles with its cluster salts. Muscle cells receive these cluster salts like a baby receives mother's milk, and the cluster salts help rid the muscles of lactic acid and toxins that have built up in them from everyday exposure. Bringing celery juice into your routine can allow for faster recovery and rebound time.

GALLSTONES

Gallstones are created in the gallbladder and the gallbladder alone. *What* creates them comes from the liver. A toxic, overburdened, sluggish, or stagnant liver is one that's filled with unusable proteins, large amounts of red blood cells, viruses and viral sludge, bacteria and bacterial sludge, and accumulated toxic substances that are foreign to the body from hundreds and hundreds of industrial chemical compounds that we breathe in, consume, or are otherwise exposed to—such as when DDT or toxic heavy metals are passed along from generation to generation.

The liver isn't meant to handle as much as this world gives it. So, unknown to medical research and science, the liver passes along some of its overload to the gallbladder, ejecting toxic material into it. The gallbladder is a cooler temperature than the liver, especially when the liver is overheated from handling too much, so when this sludge goes from the hot liver to the cooler gallbladder, stones can be forged. Whether they're bilirubin or cholesterol gallstones, they're not just bilirubin or cholesterol. They're a combination of dozens of toxins, many of which medical research and science don't yet study. Gallstones aren't clean; they're dirty.

You might have heard already that celery juice helps dissolve gallstones. Sometimes that happens with Medical Medium information: It becomes so popular that it makes its way through the world separate from the other Medical Medium healing guidance. As a result, people can end up a little lost because they don't know what else to do for their health besides drink celery juice, or they don't know when or how much to drink. Now you've traced this information back to its source. It's true—celery juice helps with existing gallstones. When sodium cluster salts enter the gallbladder, they immediately start creating divots and burrows in gallstones, filling them with holes like they're Swiss cheese so that the stones break apart and dissolve over time. Celery juice also helps slowly cleanse and revive an overburdened liver; it's one of the greatest liver detoxifiers we have, and that means it helps prevent gallstones in the first place.

(For more on gallbladder issues, see "Strep-Related Conditions.")

HAIR THINNING AND LOSS

Adrenal hormone deficiencies are commonly behind mystery hair thinning and loss. Now, the adrenal glands are complex. Medical research and science don't yet study most of the hormones they produce; medicine is still in its infancy of understanding the adrenals. In truth, they produce 56 different blends of adrenaline for different situations in life, which you can read about in *Medical Medium*. They also produce more than just adrenaline and cortisol; they produce an abundance of hormones, including reproductive ones. Celery juice is suited to help them, because it's almost as complex as the adrenal glands.

Our diets are not fortified with everything our adrenals require, so the glands can sometimes starve of essential nutrients. As you read earlier, even celery grown in poor soil will possess critical sodium cluster salts, so no matter what crop of celery it's made from, celery juice swoops in with its sodium cluster salts that specifically feed adrenal gland tissue. Once the adrenals receive celery juice's cluster salts, balance can return to the glands and they can start to produce more of their specialized plant hormones, allowing critical areas of the body such as hair follicles to receive the messages they need. The return of the hormones acts almost like plant food for the follicles, stimulating them to allow for hair growth.

People will often notice that when they're under less intense stress and in a happier place in life for long enough, they eventually experience less hair loss and maybe even new hair growth. That's because the adrenals are in a more stable place, allowing them to support the hair follicles. When we're under great stress, it's the opposite: adrenaline and cortisol can saturate hair follicles, causing bouts of hair loss for many people in this position. We can't always control what's coming at us in life. Celery juice offers the adrenals and, by extension, the hair follicles support through both harder and happier times.

HEADACHES AND MIGRAINES

People get headaches and migraines for different reasons. There are too many to share them all here, so we'll explore a choice few. (For more, see the migraines chapter in *Medical Medium*.) Rest assured, celery juice addresses all of the various root causes of headaches and migraines.

Migraines especially are still a mystery to medical research and science—millions suffer from them without understanding why. One reason for migraines is inflammation of the phrenic, vagus, and trigeminal nerves caused by neurotoxins produced by the shingles virus. (As I shared in *Medical Medium*, there are over 30 varieties of shingles; it's more common than anyone realizes.) Celery juice is an anti-inflammatory for these critical nerves, soothing, rejuvenating, and revitalizing them with its precious trace minerals from inside its sodium cluster salts. Celery juice also binds onto the neurotoxins and neutralizes their injurious properties that otherwise tend to aggravate nerves. That is, celery juice weakens their toxic nature and helps stop them from being detrimental. As a result, the phrenic, vagus, and trigeminal nerves become less sensitive to the shingles neurotoxins—they're practically shielded by celery juice's sodium cluster salts.

Another cause of migraines and head-aches is the presence of toxic heavy metals inside brain cells. Toxic heavy metal depos-its, such as those of mercury and aluminum, prompt the brain to run hot because they create blocks inside the brain that impede natural electricity flow. Instead of travel-ing freely through brain tissue, electrical impulses end up ricocheting, and not only does this heat up the brain, it means that it takes more energy for someone to process information, think, and generally function. Celery juice feeds every single brain cell, offering each one the proper nourishment to help override toxic heavy metals so that electricity can freely flow across neurons. It also enhances neurotransmitter chemicals, allowing the brain to function at its optimum level even in the face of toxic heavy metals.

Often people experience migraines and headaches due to chronic dehydration and a lack of oxygen from dirty blood. This is the result of a stagnant, sluggish liver and a high-fat diet saturating the bloodstream with an abundance of fat that pushes away oxygen and leads to minimal oxygen levels inside certain organs such as the brain. Celery juice helps disperse fats in the bloodstream, cleaning and purifying the blood while also clearing the liver of troublemakers that have accumulated there, since the liver is the main filter of the body. Revitalizing the liver brings back one of its critical chemical functions that I call the *camel effect*: taking precious water molecules from the healthy foods we eat such as apples and using it to revive "dead" water from dehydrating sources such as coffee, black tea, and soft drinks. (Read more in *Liver Rescue*.) Celery juice itself also helps us hydrate; it's the ultimate electrolyte source that helps enhance water already in the body and bloodstream, making it more vital and lowering the chronic dehydration that millions walk around with, unnoticed by medical professionals.

Celery juice also helps with stress-related, emotion-related, and tension headaches and migraines that result from the adrenaline of our chronic fight-or-flight daily lives going to the brain. Since celery juice strengthens the adrenals and neutralizes toxic adrenaline, it helps head off (so to speak) these adrenaline-surge headaches.

HEART PALPITATIONS, ECTOPIC HEARTBEATS, AND ARRHYTHMIA

If you're experiencing heart palpita-tions, ectopic heartbeats, or an arrhythmia where there isn't an obvious heart condi-tion, clogged artery, or other explanation that a cardiologist can hang their hat on, you might have heard that your issue is hormonal or genetic. Those aren't true answers. What those labels mean is that your skipped beats, heart flutters, or abnormal heartbeats are a mystery to your physician. What's really responsible is a jelly-like substance released from the liver that gathers in the mitral valve, aortic valve, or tricuspid valve and makes the heart valve (or valves) sticky. When you drink celery juice, it goes to the root cause of this sticky jelly: pathogens such as the Epstein-Barr virus.

EBV lives in most everyone's liver, and its waste matter—in the form of byproduct and viral corpses—is what creates this jelly-like substance. The jelly tends to accumulate in the liver over years, and then one day may build up to the point that some of it starts to escape. When this happens, the heart draws up the substance from the liver through the hepatic veins, at which point it can begin slightly gumming up heart valves. This can cause them to get slightly stuck, which can give you the sense of a missed heartbeat, a jump in the chest, a heartbeat that goes up to your throat, and so on. The jelly isn't as serious as plaque; it's not dangerous. It is still worth addressing, since it signals liver issues that could turn more urgent.

Celery juice combats mystery heart flutters by breaking apart this sludge when it enters the liver. The juice also improves the liver's ability to release undiscovered chemical compounds that act as degreasing agents (which I mentioned in *Liver Rescue*) to help disperse the jelly. Further, celery juice weakens the virus (such as EBV) that's responsible so that it ends up producing less viral waste and therefore minimizing buildup in the first place. Celery juice also helps with the jelly-like sludge that's already reached the heart. Its mineral salts travel through the bloodstream and enter the heart valves, where it can loosen and break down the substance and send it on its way.

HIGH CHOLESTEROL

Anything to do with cholesterol has everything to do with the liver. Any kind of cholesterol problem developing is a sign of an early liver condition developing. The liver produces, controls, organizes, and stores cholesterol. So when the liver gets sluggish, stagnant, and toxic over the years—which will go undetected at the doctor's office— and its functions start to break down, cholesterol readings can start to change. This may happen long before tests show elevated liver enzymes, so no one will realize this has anything to do with the liver.

Have you ever wondered how someone who eats the poorest diet can get back perfectly fine cholesterol readings? That's a person whose liver is not maxed out yet. Then you could have someone with a seemingly healthy diet who's diagnosed with a cholesterol condition because readings are heading in a direction the physician doesn't like. That's a person whose liver is starting to flag from being overloaded for too long. Everyone's liver has a different state of being. Some are filled with pathogens such as the Epstein-Barr virus and strep. Some are filled with both pathogens and toxins such as toxic heavy metals, pesticides, herbicides, fungicides, pharmaceuticals, plastics, and other petroleum products. When the liver's storage is at capacity, that's when its ability to process, convert, create, store, and develop cholesterol starts to diminish.

Far more powerful than any statin can ever be, celery juice goes to the root cause of cholesterol conditions: it heads to the liver. There, it helps flush, clean, and purify poisons, toxins, and pathogens. It restores and revives damaged liver lobules while its sodium cluster salts reduce viral and bacterial loads. These cluster salts also revitalize the liver's multiple functions related to cholesterol and improve the strength of the bile that the liver produces—and stronger bile helps break down fats.

HYPERTENSION (HIGH BLOOD PRESSURE)

Celery juice is an equalizer for blood pressure. While we're going to delve into high blood pressure here, know that just because celery juice can lower blood pressure for those with hypertension, that doesn't mean that you should avoid celery juice if you're dealing with low blood pressure. Celery juice meets you wherever you are. If it's low, it helps elevate it. If it's in a healthy range, it helps keep it stable. And if it's high . . . well, that's what we're about to examine.

High blood pressure is a mystery to medical research and science when a cardiologist can't find recognizable heart disease, vascular blockages, or arteriosclerosis. It's undiscovered that the liver is really what's responsible for hypertension that can't be explained by obvious sources—specifically, a stagnant, sluggish liver that's filled with toxins. Over the years, the liver becomes overburdened because it's part of the body's filtration system, collecting everything that shouldn't be in our bodies and holding on to it to try to keep us safe. Fresh, clean blood is supposed to leave the liver. When the liver becomes too taxed, though, it starts letting out dirty blood that's filled with toxins. The heart has to work 10 to 50 times harder to create suction to draw this thicker blood up from the clogged filter of the liver. That's what causes hypertension. This flies under the radar of medical testing because there isn't yet a diagnostic tool to detect a sluggish liver, or even an awareness that this precursor to fatty liver exists.

Celery juice helps free the liver of the poisons and toxins that clog it, making the organ less sluggish and stagnant. Its sodium cluster salts disperse toxic substances from the liver and also from the bloodstream, acting as a gentle, safe, body-approved blood thinning agent that breaks apart clustered toxins and unproductive fats (which are the majority of fats that float around in our bloodstream) so blood can flow more freely. The sodium cluster salts also feed the heart, strengthening it so it doesn't have to suffer from being overworked. Consumed on a regular basis, celery juice can keep working away at clearing up toxic debris from inside the liver so that eventually, the liver is releasing pure, clean blood so the heart doesn't have to overexert itself.

INSOMNIA

One cause of insomnia is emotional disturbance, whether from excess stress, loss, heartbreak, confrontation, being misunderstood, or an unresolved matter in life. Going through these experiences and losing sleep burns up neurotransmitter chemicals rapidly. When that's the case, celery juice provides the ultimate restoration of neurotransmitter chemicals. Now, sodium is a critical part of neurotransmitter chemicals. The sodium in celery juice is an entirely different make and model from what you get in other sources, and it serves as the ultimate neurotransmitter chemical component. Not to mention that bound to celery juice's sodium cluster salts are dozens of trace minerals to help your brain, too. By replenishing neurotransmitter chemicals, celery juice helps sustain you through times of turmoil.

Another reason why people can't sleep is chronic viral infection. The common virus Epstein-Barr excretes a tremendous amount of neurotoxins, which can travel through the bloodstream, enter the brain, and weaken neurotransmitters, causing sleep disturbances. Celery juice's sodium cluster salts help deactivate, disarm, and neutralize these neurotoxins, making them less damaging to neurotransmitter chemicals. Consuming celery juice long term helps break

down and destroy the virus that's producing the sleep-disturbing neurotoxins in the first place.

Insomnia can also result from problems with the liver. An unhappy, sluggish, stagnant liver that's filled with toxic byproduct can spasm during the night, waking you up out of sleep even if you can't feel the spasming. Once up, if you have to visit the bathroom or your mind starts to race, it can be tough to fall back to sleep. Celery juice helps disarm and purge the liver of toxins as well as destroy viruses in the liver that can create even more toxins there, and that helps bring the liver back to life while soothing it from liver hypertension. A calmed liver translates to fewer spasms and less disrupted sleep.

Some people don't sleep because of a sensitive nervous system overall. Nerve aches and pains, restless legs syndrome, twitches, spasms, and nerve weakness often don't allow people to sleep properly. The same goes for people diagnosed with neurological conditions such as ME/CFS or Lyme disease. Celery juice's sodium cluster salts are the most powerful electrolytes Planet Earth has to offer at this time from any food—electrolytes that help protect the central nervous system so people can experience alleviation of the neurological conditions and symptoms and autoimmune disorders that so many experience.

Oftentimes, people can't sleep because of sensitive intestinal linings due to inflammation. This means that food traveling through the gut at night can awaken someone constantly. As with liver spasms, this can occur on a level that the person doesn't even feel; it could seem like they wake up for no reason. Celery juice improves digestion on all levels. For example, it strengthens hydrochloric acid so that proteins digest better. It restores worn-out intestinal linings' natural sandpaper-like texture so they can better grip, process, and round up fiber. And because celery juice helps restore intestinal nerve endings, which receive messages to create peristaltic action, it allows for smoother peristalsis. This all translates to better sleep.

JOINT PAIN AND ARTHRITIS

When someone is dealing with arthritis, there could be a couple of different issues going on. For one, calcifications can develop over the years, building up and clinging around joints and joint sockets, and these bring wear and tear to cartilage. They can also be accompanied by many different toxins and poisons such as toxic heavy metals settling in joint areas all through the body—the result of a liver that's been sluggish and stagnant long term. Toxins plus calcifications lead to what many experience as the typical arthritis that accompanies aging. Bone spurs that lower someone's quality of life can also develop over time. These are basically bone nodules that develop from toxic exposure, too.

Celery juice helps lubricate joints and cartilage, strengthen tendons and connective tissue around joints, and reduce the nerve inflammation that can occur in joint areas as well. Celery juice has the unique ability to break up and disperse calcium deposits—which is the same unique ability it has to dissolve gallstones, kidney stones, adhesions, and scar tissue. It's part of what makes celery juice so miraculous. Much of its ability to disassemble calcium deposits a fragment at a time, releasing them back into the bloodstream to be carried out of the body, has to do with its alkalinity factor. Celery juice is extremely alkalizing once it enters the body. This is not to be confused with sources that are highly alkaline outside the body, such as high-pH water, which is actually not productive for the body's pH. Read more in *Liver Rescue*. When celery juice enters the stomach, it starts to alter rapidly, becoming far more alkaline than it was to begin with. This is part of how it reduces the pains of arthritis.

For insight into rheumatoid arthritis and psoriatic arthritis, turn back to page 35.

KIDNEY DISEASE AND KIDNEY STONES

Kidney injury is what leads to kidney dysfunction and disease. Now, kidney injury can come in different forms. One form is toxic injury from pharmaceuticals, recreational drugs, toxic heavy metals, pesticides, herbicides, and solvents.

By far the most common cause of kidney disease is pathogenic injury, which results when viruses or bacteria enter the kidney via blood vessels or the urinary tract. The most common viruses that cause this are HHV-6, HHV-7, and EBV—and they're under the radar of medical research and science as far as kidney disease goes. When a virus inflames a kidney, a physician will often mistakenly believe that it's the immune system attacking the gland. When it comes to kidney tumors and cysts, whether cancerous or benign, viruses play a role in creating them, too. In the case of bacterial kidney infections, strep is a common cause; it's also responsible for urinary tract infections (UTIs) that turn into severe kidney infections.

And then there's food injury. Diets high in protein shorten the life of the kidneys. The popularity of high-protein diets is quite extraordinary considering that even medical research and science are aware that people with even a slight kidney issue cannot consume too much protein. High-protein diets are high in fat, too, and that combination creates a lot of wear and tear on the kidneys, bogging them down, tiring them out, and setting the stage for pathogens, or any of the other injury sources we just examined, to push the kidneys over the edge.

Especially if you're going through dialysis or another complicated kidney procedure, speak to your doctor before applying anything to your life, including celery juice. If your doctor is comfortable with it, know that celery juice is gentle on the kidneys and in small dosages can be very helpful. As with any kidney problem or disease, large dosages of anything are not ideal, whether large dosages of medicine, animal protein, plant-based protein, or certain supplements. Even with celery juice, we still need to be respectful and mindful that

when kidneys are in a weakened, problematic state, more isn't necessarily best. Small dosages of celery juice can provide those suffering with kidney disease with trace minerals, vitamin C, and some sodium cluster salts to fight off pathogens responsible for most kidney dysfunction. Small dosages of celery juice also help rejuvenate the kidneys from toxic damage caused by sources such as chemical exposure or long-term exposure to excess protein. The adrenals struggle when the kidneys weaken, and celery juice's plant hormones help restore the adrenal glands, too.

Celery juice also helps diminish and dissolve kidney stones, which are produced from high-protein, high-fat diets. Kidney stones can be protein-based or calcium-based or even some of both. Celery juice creates pits and divots on the stones, which is what allows them to break down and dissolve. It can also be a great kidney stone preventative. While it's not a complete assurance that you won't develop kidney stones if you're still eating a high-fat diet, it can help counteract some of the effects of the protein and fat overload.

LOSS OF LIBIDO

When everything else checks out okay and a woman's sex drive disappears mysteriously, weakened adrenals (which can go unnoticed by a physician) are usually the cause. The trace minerals bound to celery juice's sodium cluster salts revitalize adrenal tissue, infusing it and strengthening its ability to produce the particular adrenaline that's released by the adrenals during sex.

Men can have a strong sex drive even with weak adrenals. What's often responsible for a man's loss of libido are weakened neurotransmitter chemicals in certain areas of the brain, elevated toxic heavy metals, or both. Celery juice helps restore neurons and brain tissue, replaces neurotransmitter chemicals, and helps loosen heavy metals and prepare them for export out of the brain.

METABOLISM PROBLEMS

"Metabolism" does not mean what we've come to believe it does. As I uncovered in *Thyroid Healing*, a slow metabolism is not truly behind anybody's symptoms or conditions; it never was and it never will be. That's because the term *metabolism* describes the discovery of our being alive, that our blood is pumping and our body is functioning. A "slow metabolism" does not give us an answer to what can truly go wrong in the body to create a condition such as weight gain. That said, "metabolism" has become the law of the land, heralded as an explanation for people's struggles. So if we want to go along with it, then yes, in a manner of speaking, drinking celery juice speeds up your metabolism. It can indeed help you lose weight.

The true cause of what's called a slow metabolism is a sluggish liver. It's as simple as that, and helping out your liver is what helps you lose weight. What's complicated

is this: Our livers are filled with a variety of what I call troublemakers that we encounter in our everyday lives. These include pesticides, fungicides, herbicides, toxic heavy metals, synthetic chemicals, viruses, bacteria, plastics, and even toxic hormones such as excess adrenaline. When the liver gets clogged up with these plus the fat cells from a high-fat, high-protein diet, the troublemakers slow it down, making the liver sluggish, causing someone to develop a pre-fatty or dysfunctional liver. As a result, the fat storage inside the liver gets overcrowded, so the body starts to store fats in other areas.

Celery juice revives liver cells by flushing out these various toxins and also helping dissolve and disperse fat cells—essentially, celery juice cleans out your liver, removing a variety of toxins and reducing viral loads. This awakens the liver, bringing it back to life, and when your liver improves, so does everything else in your body. Every organ becomes cleaner. The blood and lymphatic system even become cleaner and less toxic. If that's what you want to call improving your metabolism, then you're welcome to do that. At the same time, know what's going on beneath the surface: the liver is improving thanks to celery juice.

MTHFR GENE MUTATIONS AND METHYLATION ISSUES

Celery juice can reduce the elevated homocysteine levels associated with patients diagnosed with MTHFR (methylenetetrahydrofolate reductase) gene mutations. Homocysteine levels rise when the liver is chronically inflamed, and celery juice aids the liver by recharging, rejuvenating, and replenishing it, while also cleansing the liver of the high elevation of toxins that tend to inhabit it. A common type of toxin in the liver comes from viral waste. When viruses such as EBV are active in the body, they excrete debris in the liver, and as these toxins build up long term, they wreak havoc by inflaming the organ. Celery juice neutralizes these toxins, both in the liver and throughout the bloodstream. Even if someone doesn't have an elevated homocysteine level, the cause of what's labeled as an MTHFR gene mutation is the same: a chronic viral load, whether low grade or elevated, inside the liver, causing the organ to become overburdened and weakened. The inflammation here is not just in the liver; it can be throughout the whole body, even without homocysteine markers. Inflammation rises when viral toxins are flooding the bloodstream, and that's what triggers a positive on an MTHFR gene mutation test—which is really an inflammation test.

Celery juice's sodium cluster salts help neutralize and lower the amount of viral toxins floating through the bloodstream and elevating inflammation. Celery juice helps flush these toxins out of the liver, bloodstream, and kidneys. The folate in celery juice is also critical for people struggling with methylation issues and MTHFR gene mutation diagnoses, because this form of folate is so easy to convert for a weak, struggling liver that's not methylating properly. Once the liver is healthier from long-term celery juice, it can start to methylate properly again, which is vital, since receiving vitamins and other nutrients from the intestinal tract, converting them, sometimes storing them, and releasing them into the bloodstream in more bioavailable form is one of the liver's most important functions. This can lower inflammation throughout the body and reverse an MTHFR gene mutation test result.

If this sounds confusing, know that it has happened for many: an initial gene mutation test has come back positive, and then after applying the right healing techniques, a follow-up test has shown that someone no longer has a gene mutation. It tends to baffle physicians. The truth is that once you recover the liver using larger quantities of celery juice and other healing approaches that you can read about in the Medical Medium series, you can clean up what's really a misinterpreted and ambiguous diagnosis. If this new line of thinking has you rattled, look into *Liver Rescue* so you can discover the full truth about MTHFR gene mutations.

NEUROLOGICAL SYMPTOMS

Tightness in the Chest, Trembling Hands, Twitches and Spasms, Muscle Weakness, Tingles and Numbness, Restless Legs, Restlessness, Weakness of the Limbs, Muscle Spasms, Aches and Pains

Individuals who experience neurological symptoms for no discernible reason such as injury have something in common: they're struggling with a viral load, often from the Epstein-Barr virus. There are over 60 varieties of EBV, and at least one strain of it sits in most everyone's liver. For many people, the virus is dormant, so they'll never know it's there. For many others, it's active, though working under the radar of medical research and science, so they'll still never know it's there—even though it's causing multiple symptoms or conditions that affect them every day.

For a virus such as EBV to actively cause health problems, it needs fuel. Among its favorite fuels are toxic heavy metals such as mercury. The liver is a collecting place for troublemakers like heavy metals, and there are usually plenty of them to be had there. When EBV consumes the heavy metal, it excretes it in much more potent form: as a neurotoxin. Viral neurotoxins are, as the name suggests, toxic to nerves, and they're behind millions and millions of people's neurological suffering.

The viral strain and level of toxic heavy metals (mostly mercury and aluminum) that someone has determine their individual experience and symptomology. How toxic is the neurotoxin that the virus is expelling? How aggressive is the virus that's reproducing itself as it gobbles down heavy metals and other forms of viral fuel? Once excreted, neurotoxins tend to leave the liver (or any other place where the virus has produced them in the body), float through the bloodstream, and eventually enter the brain or land on nerves throughout the body. When viral neurotoxins land on nerves, they inflame the nerves, which leads to neurological symptoms. If the neurotoxins land specifically on nerves in the legs, arms, shoulders, or spine, it can result in muscle heaviness, weakness, or tiredness in one limb or more. They can also cause a more general neurological fatigue, where the whole body feels heavy and weighted down, as though something is pinning down and compromising the person. When neurotoxins enter the brain, very similar symptoms occur. Messages to the arms and limbs can be compromised, leading to fatigue and weakness on one or both sides of the body. (Read more on neurological fatigue in "Fatigue," page 58.)

Viral neurotoxins can be so potent that they trigger muscle spasms and twitches, too. This happens when nerves are getting signals fired off from the brain that something is in the way or agitating neurons in the brain tissue. Neurotoxins are that "something." When a neuron becomes saturated with neurotoxins, electricity in the brain trying to travel across that neuron instead ricochets or short-circuits when it hits the neurotoxins. These electrical misfires can cause mild bouts of brain inflammation. Electrical impulses have a difficult time traveling through inflamed brain tissue; they're often forced to detour and find unusual pathways across other neurons—and this can create feelings in the limbs of twitches, spasms, and even unexplainable aches and pains in places where there's no injury present.

Tingles and numbness can result from brain tissue that's saturated with neurotoxins as well, although these symptoms mainly occur when nerves in the limbs, neck, or other spots in the body are slightly inflamed from neurotoxins landing on them.

Trembling hands often happen because someone has higher levels of mercury in both the liver and the brain—and because EBV is feeding off the mercury, creating more potent neurotoxins, which end up inflaming nerves close to the brain. This inflammation tends to happen sporadically due to moments when the virus proliferates or finds new deposits of mercury on which to feed.

Often people with Lyme disease face neurological symptoms. This, too, is viral—it's not bacterial. (If this upsets, angers, or alarms you because it differs from what you've heard before about Lyme, please read the chapter "Lyme Disease" in my first book, *Medical Medium*, so you can protect yourself with the truth.)

For everything we've just explored, it's celery juice to the rescue. To begin with, celery juice feeds every cell in the body with its sodium cluster salts, helping restore them so they can function at their optimum level. When nerves throughout the body become inflamed, impeded, hindered, damaged, or broken from neurotoxins, they require electrolytes like the elevated form that celery juice possesses. This allows neurons, brain tissue, and neurotransmitter chemicals to restore themselves and helps reduce brain and cell inflammation caused by neurotoxins from viruses such as EBV. At the same time, celery juice's sodium cluster salts allow your nerves to defend themselves against neurotoxins and the allergic reaction that they cause. Celery juice also flushes neurotoxins from the brain and the rest of the nervous system and neutralizes them so they lose the aggressive, toxic power that's responsible for these symptoms. After rendering the neurotoxins nontoxic, cluster salts bind onto them and carry them out of the body, not to mention that the cluster salts help kill off the virus itself.

OBSESSIVE-COMPULSIVE DISORDER (OCD)

One cause of OCD is emotional injury. Chronic illness, for example, can cause confusing symptoms and a long-term struggle to be heard, and that can lead to emotional injury. Many other difficult life experiences can affect our brain's emotional centers, too.

OCD can also be caused by toxic heavy metals such as mercury and aluminum. Deposits of these metals inside the brain can block electrical impulses meant to travel across neurons into tissue. When the impulses instead hit heavy metal deposits or heavy metal oxidative runoff, the electricity gets derailed or even bounces back across the neuron in the opposite direction. An obsessive-compulsive reaction can result. Because the metals can situate themselves in different places in the brain and in different amounts, they can lead to hundreds of varieties of OCD. This is a real physiological condition, and there's so much misinformation about it that makes OCD sufferers feel misunderstood.

Celery juice helps heal the emotional side of OCD by strengthening neurons in the emotional centers of the brain. Celery juice also holds special antioxidants that do more than the antioxidants from other foods, which help stop the oxidation and death of our human cells. The antioxidants in celery juice prevent toxic heavy metals from oxidizing, rusting, and corroding in the first place. They do this by removing the fatty deposits we develop when raised on high-fat diets—because removing these fatty deposits from metals prevents them from oxidizing further. Less oxidation of heavy metals leads to fewer symptoms of OCD. To continue the healing process, look into the Heavy Metal Detox Smoothie. You'll find a recipe for it in Chapter 8.

OVERACTIVE BLADDER (OAB)

Chronic inflammation of the bladder lining or the nerves related to the bladder is what causes OAB. Commonly, it's bacteria such as strep colonizing the bladder, eventually causing scar tissue and little divots and pits in the bladder lining. This leads to constant, chronic irritation and OAB. Viruses such as Epstein-Barr can also inflame nerves in and around the bladder. Even the pudendal and sciatic nerves can affect the bladder's sensitivity levels. The shingles virus, too, can inflame nerves in and around the bladder. Celery juice breaks down and destroys the pathogens behind OAB, whether bacterial or viral. Sodium cluster salts enter the bladder and break up bacterial colonies, loosen debris from both bacteria and viruses, protect the bladder lining so it can heal and mend, and essentially wash the bladder lining of any pathogenic byproduct. Celery juice also helps heal the nerves in and around the bladder.

PARKINSON'S DISEASE

Parkinson's is sometimes believed to be caused by a loss of the neurotransmitter chemical dopamine in the brain. This is not accurate. The lack of dopamine is not enough to create a disease or illness. Now, the lack of many different varieties of neurotransmitters, dopamine being just one, can be *part* of a cause. People with Parkinson's are suffering from a loss of multiple neurotransmitter chemicals. What causes this is neurons damaged and overrun by toxic heavy metals. In Parkinson's, the leading heavy metal is mercury. Mercury deposits oxidize quickly and release very toxic oxidative debris that starts to coat adjacent brain tissue, smothering neurons. When a neuron is smothered like this, its neurotransmitters also become saturated with the oxidative material, and they quickly diminish. So really, Parkinson's is the result of heavy metal runoff and the loss of many neurotransmitter chemicals that this causes.

The antioxidants in celery juice help stop the oxidative runoff process. With Parkinson's, it's also critical to restore neurons, and celery juice does this by infusing neurons with various trace minerals. Celery juice helps the liver formulate and methylate vitamin B_{12}, and since sodium cluster salts have the unique ability to carry nutrients to the brain at a high velocity, cluster salts carry these trace amounts of B_{12} all the way from the liver up to the brain, where it's critical for neuron growth. Long-term consumption of higher levels of celery juice can help restore diminished neurotransmitter chemicals and refurbish neurons, getting them to regrow.

If someone is already suffering from severe symptoms of Parkinson's, it will take much longer to reverse the condition. The longer oxidative discharge from toxic heavy metals has been saturating brain tissue adjacent to the heavy metal deposits, the longer it takes to restore neurons and brain tissue. Someone with a milder variety of Parkinson's has a better chance of reestablishing neurotransmitter chemicals faster and recovering more quickly. For anyone dealing with Parkinson's, consider augmenting your celery juice routine by also actively removing toxic heavy metals with a daily Heavy Metal Detox Smoothie (see Chapter 8).

POSTTRAUMATIC STRESS SYMPTOMS (PTSS, ALSO KNOWN AS POSTTRAUMATIC STRESS DISORDER, OR PTSD)

Emotional injuries of the brain result in the symptoms of posttraumatic stress. PTSS is in truth a variety of OCD. PTSS is similar to OCD in the sense that it's difficult to control, can be triggered easily and seemingly at random, and can also take milder or more extreme forms. How PTSS develops for different individuals depends on their other compromises and sensitivities. Someone who's already sensitive due to a high level of toxic heavy metals inside the brain, for example, can be more prone to PTSS. Pesticides, herbicides, and fungicides alone can actually cause PTSS. Exposure to radiation can also weaken an individual, making them more susceptible to PTSS. That's why people who are undergoing medical treatments will often develop small bouts of PTSS, whether during or after. Given the traumas present in our world, everyone struggles from at least a little bit of PTSS, whether barely identifiable or the severe type that can develop when someone has faced grave danger or physical or emotional abuse.

Celery juice is the most powerful electrolyte source available, and electrolytes have a lot to do with PTSS recovery. In PTSS, certain parts of the brain become wired in such a way that they become overactive and generate intense heat. Stimulating thoughts and emotions such as pain, fear, and guilt can keep electricity surging through emotional areas of the brain, creating a vicious cycle. It's hard to find a way to interrupt this cycle. Celery juice's nutrients provide respite by nourishing neurons, brain tissue, and glial cells and restoring neurotransmitters so that neurons don't overheat from continual fear, worry, concern, and mental images. Celery juice helps stop the meltdown-burnout process of the neurons so that people have a fighting chance of recovering from PTSS without medication. Continued use of celery juice in larger volumes can be the greatest aid for someone suffering with any variety of PTSS.

REPRODUCTIVE SYSTEM DISORDERS

If you're wondering if celery juice is good for your reproductive system, the answer is an overwhelming yes. The reproductive system is in desperate need of what celery juice possesses. Celery juice stops pathogens that are responsible for most reproductive symptoms, conditions, and diseases; removes toxins that are also partly responsible; with its cleansing power, binds onto, neutralizes, and escorts out toxic hormones (such as foreign estrogen from foods, plastics, other petrochemicals, and pharmaceuticals) that build up in the reproductive system and confuse the body; and nourishes and feeds the reproductive system on all levels, from restoring cells to balancing healthy hormones to providing nutrients and trace minerals to reproductive organs and glands. Critically, celery

juice also hydrates the reproductive system, which is a major factor in what can go wrong. The reproductive system ages faster than many other parts of the human body, and one reason for this is chronic dehydration of its cells. Celery juice helps prevent and reverse this.

Don't feel thwarted if you don't see your symptom, condition, or disease in the list that follows. Any reproductive system issue is a candidate for celery juice.

Breast Density

Breast density occurs when the liver has become toxic through the decades. An overburdened, sluggish, stagnant liver filled with a large volume of the troublemakers explored in *Liver Rescue* bog it down to the point that it's not able to act as the proper filter it once was. The lymphatic system becomes a secondary filter, which basically means that the breasts become secondary filters, with a lot of toxins accumulating there because of all the lymphatic vessels present. Years of poor diet components and everyday exposures to toxic substances find their way inside breast tissue, creating calcifications and scar tissue. We're not talking about scar tissue from breast surgery. This is scar tissue from cells not getting enough vital oxygen and nutrients.

Calcium from dairy products is a leading contributor to breast density, because the calcium settles in breast tissue. This is not a healthy calcium; it's an aggressive calcium that's antagonistic to women's health and becomes fuel for pathogens. Toxic heavy metals such as mercury and aluminum settle in the breast tissue, as well. If someone's diet is not adequately hydrating, then dehydration of breast tissue can occur slowly over time as well, keeping cells from becoming revitalized by critical living water. The Epstein-Barr virus is responsible for more advanced breast conditions and issues.

Celery juice not only cleanses and frees the liver over time, it helps cleanse the lymphatic system as well by bringing in fresh deliveries of living water filled with sodium cluster salts, trace minerals, and phytochemicals to flush out the troublemakers. Rejuvenating the lymphatic system has everything to do with cleaning up breast tissue. Celery juice's unique travel velocity and saturation rate also mean that it has the ability to find its way through dense, hardened, fibrous breast tissue all the way to the skin. Celery juice provides anti-tumor, anti-adhesion properties.

Cysts

Cysts can develop from a variety of toxins (such as toxic heavy metals, pesticides, herbicides, and fungicides) and from viruses such as Epstein-Barr. These cysts can be benign or cancerous. Many cysts are lymphatic vessel scar tissue surrounding the reproductive system that became inflamed and hardened, and maybe even calcified, due to viral infection. Celery juice helps break down these calcifications and hardened, chronic cysts. It also helps loosen up, break down, and disperse scar tissue that

can otherwise become keloids or adhesion varieties of cysts. Celery juice feeds healthy cells around cysts, too, making them stronger, which helps stop the growth of cysts that are nearby. Cysts tend to thrive energetically around toxic, unhealthy cells. When they're surrounded by healthy cells, it prevents them from thriving and expanding.

Endometriosis

Celery juice provides undiscovered phytochemical compound inhibitors to excess abnormal tissue growth. These inhibitors push back on endometrial tissue that tries to develop outside of the uterus, colon, and bladder. Abnormal tissue growth is abnormal due to the presence of toxins. Unhealthy cells develop and expand where they're not supposed to from a combination of toxic, unhealthy hormones that are foreign to the body coupled with troublemakers such as pesticides, herbicides, fungicides, toxic heavy metals (such as mercury and aluminum), and viral and bacterial byproduct and debris. Celery juice breaks up and disperses all of these toxins so they can't fuel abnormal tissue development. Combined with its inhibiting phytochemical compounds, this makes celery juice a potent tonic for endometriosis sufferers.

Fibroids

Fibroids in the uterus take various forms, with their cause unknown by medical research and science. The truth is that fibroids are sometimes caused by viruses such as Epstein-Barr and other times caused by bacteria such as strep. When it's viral, it's more of a cystic variety of fibroid, with a rounder shape. When it's bacterial, it's more like scar tissue or an adhesion inside the reproductive system. The sodium cluster salts in celery juice seek out and destroy bacteria and viruses, minimizing the pathogenic loads responsible for fibroids while also helping shrink existing fibroids.

Human Papillomavirus (HPV)

HPV has no immunity against celery juice. The virus is similar in many ways to herpetic family viruses such as EBV and shingles in that its sensitivity lies in the virus cells' outer membranes, where sodium cluster salts can attach themselves and slowly break down the virus's defense mechanisms. Regular consumption of celery juice can minimize growth of HPV and protect the cervix from developing scar tissue and what doctors often think are compromised cells due to HPV exposure that could eventually lead to cancer. Once you have the weapons—such as celery juice—to fight it, and you're avoiding foods that can feed the virus (more in Chapter 8), you have set the stage for protecting yourself from and even eliminating HPV over time.

Infertility

For the majority of women suffering from infertility, it's a medical mystery. Everything seems to check out okay at the doctor's office, and no one can explain why they are having trouble conceiving or carrying a healthy baby to term. I call this *low battery.* Many factors from the past can trigger a low reproductive system battery. Contraceptive use is one of them; it trains the reproductive system to operate in shutdown mode. Celery juice can revive a reproductive system that's been trained for years not to produce, because it revives cells and organs and removes toxins that contraceptives have left behind, giving the system a fresh start. Celery juice also provides plant hormones that the human body can adapt to recharge glands and organs that produce healthy hormones, including the adrenals and other endocrine glands and the liver, which is another hormone producer. This can prompt the reproductive system to normalize and balance, putting it in good working order to remind it that it can bear fruit.

For male infertility, celery juice provides a highly assimilable form of trace mineral zinc and other critical trace minerals that can be used to instantly bring down inflammation of the prostate gland. The prostate is susceptible to low-grade chronic infections of strep, other bacteria, and EBV, whether from sexual or nonsexual activity. This potent zinc prevents them from wreaking havoc in the prostate and causing prostatitis.

Many men suffer from weakened kidneys, and these easily fly under the radar at the doctor's office. We're not talking kidney disease, only weakness. Weakened kidneys in men lead to weakened reproductive systems. Depending on the stage of kidney weakness, it can lead to backaches that just seem like sore muscles, or sleeping issues, irritability and crankiness, or body odor. When the kidneys are suffering, the reproductive system breaks down and loses its vitality faster, sometimes even becoming diseased. Celery juice provides the TLC that weary kidneys need, and when celery juice strengthens the kidneys, a man's reproductive system is more protected and can recover more quickly.

(For more on infertility, see the chapter "Fertility and Our Future" in *Life-Changing Foods*.)

Menopause Symptoms

The symptoms of perimenopause, menopause, and postmenopause are not caused by an aging reproductive system. They're caused by an aging liver. When the liver becomes sluggish, stagnant, and toxic—which coincidentally happens to the majority of women in their late 30s to late 40s—symptoms such as hot flashes, night sweats, irritability, fatigue, depression, anxiety, and loss of libido can start to appear. When the liver is filled with viral byproduct, viral neurotoxins, and viruses themselves such as Epstein-Barr, heart palpitations can start to occur, too, as viral waste is released into the bloodstream. For many individuals, the symptoms associated with menopause can be arrested simply with celery juice alone. It helps bring back and revitalize the liver, lower viral loads, lower viral toxins, and remove other poisons that have caused the liver to become sluggish and stagnant over the decades. A cleaner, healthier liver

means relief from symptoms labeled as menopause.

For much more on menopause, see *Medical Medium* and *Thyroid Healing*.

Pelvic Inflammatory Disease (PID)

PID is the result of *Streptococcus* bacteria in the reproductive system. Celery helps over time via its sodium cluster salts entering the reproductive system through the blood and lymph vessels, helping to destroy strep once it's there. Cluster salts also deliver celery juice's signature vitamin C to boost the reproductive immune system.

Polycystic Ovarian Syndrome (PCOS)

PCOS is caused by the Epstein-Barr virus creating fluid-filled cysts and other ovarian injuries. Celery juice helps stop this. Its sodium cluster salts break down and destroy EBV and then help detox the ovaries of their viral toxins and debris.

STREP-RELATED CONDITIONS

Most people, when they think of *Streptococcus* bacteria, think of strep throat. That's not all that strep causes. There's a host of other conditions that occur in people's lives, whether at earlier or later ages, that are the result of low-grade chronic strep inside the body. Strep is a type of bacteria that has built up its platform and strength in our environment and world due to the overuse of antibiotics. That's right:

antibiotics have shaped and sculpted strep into what it is today. So many different groups, strains, and mutations of strep exist that medical research and science cannot keep up with them.

Strep throat is just one indication of strep. If you're someone who took antibiotics early in life for a cough, flu, or childhood ear infection, that could have set the stage for future episodes of strep-related illnesses. What if you're someone who's never taken antibiotics before in your life? Does that mean you weren't exposed to them? I'm sorry to say no. Antibiotics are in our water supply, they're in our food, and they're passed from generations before us through our family bloodline. As a result, almost everybody lives with one or multiple varieties of strep in their system. It's a common bug that we all live with. When you have celery juice in your daily regimen, though, you don't have to be a prisoner to strep.

Celery juice is the ultimate strep fighter. Its sodium cluster salts destroy strep on contact throughout the body, and that makes it amazing for the many conditions you're about to examine. Celery juice's vitamin C helps boost the immune system against strep-related illnesses. Its multitudes of trace minerals help strengthen tissue and organs from the damage that strep bacteria colonies can cause.

Healing from strep is one reason why so many people are healing from so many conditions—because it's involved in so much. If you're young, you might have only experienced acne, strep throat, or an ear infection—which probably doesn't feel like an "only" since each condition can be so disruptive. As individuals enter their 20s and 30s, they may start to develop additional strep-related issues: sinusitis, even more strep throat, a UTI, a yeast infection. As time goes on, maybe someone receives a diagnosis of SIBO or *Candida*. What no one ever tells them—because no one realizes—is that all of these seemingly unrelated, years-apart diagnoses trace back to strep, some of which has been in the system for a long, long time. The bacteria tend to hide out long term inside the liver, building colonies and causing more and more trouble as the liver becomes more weakened, sluggish, and stagnant. Celery juice gives you more control over this bug than ever before.

Acne

As I shared in *Liver Rescue*, acne is a sign of early wars in life that go undocumented. Those early wars usually began with strep causing one of the issues in this list. As a result, antibiotics entered the body—prescribed, for example, for an ear infection—and counter to what anyone intended, those antibiotics lent strength to strep. In some cases, antibiotics didn't even enter the system through pharmaceuticals; someone consumed them through food or water or inherited them through the bloodline. In whatever form antibiotics arrived, they gave strep a chance to thrive.

Medical research and science believe that acne is a hormone-based condition.

They're mistaken. Acne tends to accompany hormonal shifts such as puberty and menstruation because the immune system lowers dramatically at these times, allowing strep to take advantage and create a condition such as acne. Acne isn't caused by clogged pores, either. While sure, a clogged pore can cause a pimple here and there, a series of aggressive cysts is a sign of a strep infection sitting in the liver and traveling up through the lymphatic system to the dermis searching for food. We all hear about the oily skin that usually goes along with acne. That sebum oil is produced to try to stop the strep bacteria from causing harm.

The sodium cluster salts in celery juice help disperse sebum oil, exposing strep and destroying it while at the same time allowing your immune system to destroy strep, too. Lymphocytes (a type of white blood cell) feed on the trace minerals in celery juice and get a boost from its vitamin C so they can enter the dermis and defend you from strep creating cystic acne there. Taking foods such as dairy, gluten, and eggs out of the diet also reduces acne because these are favorite foods of strep, and keeping them out of the system helps starve strep. While celery juice is destroying strep in your liver and lymphatic system and strengthening lymphocytes, it helps flush out remnants of any toxic foods you might have been consuming that were lending fuel to strep. This, too, helps lead to clearer skin.

Appendicitis

Appendicitis often occurs from food poisoning. For that to happen, the appendix has to be weakened in the first place. People can also develop appendicitis without food poisoning. Either way, the appendix area is harboring colonies of strep. Why is it there? The immune system is highly active in the appendix area; the appendix acts as a lure to bacteria such as strep so that the immune system can destroy them. If too much strep is present in the body, though, for too many years, this can cause wear and tear on the appendix. Eventually, it can lead to an acute rupture or inflammatory condition.

Celery juice is amazing for the appendix. When celery juice is near, strep tends to run from the appendix. Celery juice enters into the appendix via the colon and also from outside the colon, via the lymphatic vessels, helping soothe and heal an inflamed appendix. It also helps destroy strep bacteria, ridding it and even repelling it from the area.

Diverticulitis

Diverticulitis can occur from one of two different types of bacteria: *E. coli* or *Streptococcus*. For the most part, strep is the more common cause, creating more long-term inflammation that leads to diverticulitis. Strep-related diverticulitis normally occurs later in life, because it can take many years for strep to proliferate past the small intestinal tract and start building pockets in the colon. Often, the strep in the system has also caused at least one of the other issues in this list, which has led to the use of antibiotics as early as childhood, and that has allowed the strep to grow and strengthen over time.

Normally, it's not an aggressive variety of strep that's behind diverticulitis. It's usually one of the milder varieties that has colonized there for decades. Sometimes strep and *E. coli* do work together, kind of like different insects inside a tree burrow, each of them finding different foods they like, working together as they create those little pockets known as diverticula.

Celery juice is a miracle for diverticulitis, because its sodium cluster salts tend to go into the diverticula—the little pits and divots and potholes that developed inside the colon. Celery juice cleans and flushes out the strep- and *E. coli*-filled pockets and eliminates these canker sores, allowing the colon lining to start to mend and heal.

Ear Infections

Almost all ear infections are strep-caused. This is why when antibiotics are prescribed for ear infections, they're not always effective, especially if someone has taken antibiotics for an ear infection before—because strep tends to build immunity to antibiotics, especially with constant use of them. Most ear infections start in childhood. Taking antibiotics for them can lead strep to become resistant early in life, and that can lead to more problems with the other strep-related conditions in this list as a person gets older.

When strep is inside the ear in any way, it means it's in the lymphatic system. Celery juice's sodium cluster salts are able to enter the lymphatic system quickly, easily, and efficiently—within hours of consumption. These cluster salts seek and destroy strep they find there to reduce the risk of future ear infections.

Gallbladder Issues

Gallbladder infections that are not caused by gallstones are strep-related infections. Strep tends to hide out and camp in the liver. It also likes to be in the duodenum and the rest of the small intestinal tract. This all means that strep can find its way to the gallbladder through the bile duct system. There, strep tends to feed on gunk and sludge—toxic chemicals and even the pulverized debris of toxic food—that build up in the gallbladder. Celery juice helps break up and send away that sludge. When celery juice enters the liver, it pushes sodium cluster salts through the hepatic ducts into the gallbladder, and from there, celery juice can then dissolve the gunk buildup while killing off strep that's in both the bile duct and the gallbladder.

People who've had their gallbladders removed, when they hear that celery juice can increase bile production and strength, sometimes worry that this means they should avoid celery juice. It's quite the opposite. When you're missing your gallbladder, you still want your liver strong, and you still want it to produce bile. If your liver is weak, it affects everything else in your body; your liver getting sick from certain toxins stuck inside can make you sick down the road.

The only reason that a liver starts increasing bile production is because the liver is expelling these toxins and getting healthier and stronger in the process. A healthier, stronger liver means you won't become nutrient deficient. It means your liver can provide other parts of your body with nutrients to keep you alive longer. It means you won't age as fast. It means you can better avoid cholesterol issues, high blood pressure, and heart disease. Celery juice leads to increased bile strength only because that's part of the whole process of rebuilding the liver, not because it's a worrisome side effect. So avoiding celery juice because someone doesn't want stronger, increased bile is like avoiding it because they want their liver to stay weakened and sick. Nobody really wants that.

The truth is that celery juice is critical for people who've had gallbladder surgery. As much as anyone, people missing their gallbladders need clean, strong livers. These people usually have a hard time breaking down and digesting fats, and not only does celery juice help indirectly by aiding the liver, it also helps directly break down and disperse fats, offering relief to someone who's living life without a gallbladder.

Sinusitis

Many cases of sinusitis are acute, accompanying an illness such as the flu.

While recovering from the flu, you can produce a tremendous amount of mucus, and that mucus can become difficult to expel as the body keeps producing volumes of it to protect you from the flu virus causing damage to your sinus canals.

Chronic sinusitis is a bit different. Here, strep bacteria are camping out in the sinus cavities, sometimes for a lifetime. Ear, nose, and throat doctors often offer sinus surgery in which they scrape off scar tissue from the sinuses as a method of relief. This almost never works long term. Usually people still suffer from chronic sinusitis post-surgery. That's because it's unknown that what's really causing the sinus migraines, sinus mucus, sinus discharge, and sinus pain are high levels of strep bacteria, and those don't go away with surgery. Often, people with sinusitis have consumed antibiotics along the way, and that has contributed to strep's strength in their system.

Long-term use of celery juice is very beneficial for sinusitis. Because the sinuses are so tied to the lymphatic vessels, and the lymphatic system is one of the greatest delivery systems for celery juice's chemical compounds, the healing benefits of celery juice can reach the sinuses with ease. Celery juice's chemical compounds also find their way to the sinus cavities through the bloodstream, offering support from another angle. Once again, it's celery juice's sodium cluster salts and vitamin C that offer the immune system the tools they need to help fight off strep.

Small Intestinal Bacterial Overgrowth (SIBO), *Candida*, and Intestinal Cramping

Candida became a popular diagnosis years ago. The truth is that this form of fungus is not the problem everyone thinks it is. *Candida* is not a hazardous fungus; it's actually helpful. It accumulates, prospers, and grows where bacteria are present—and it's the bacteria that are problematic. Elevations of *Candida* are warning signs there's an invader present: that elevations of strep are building, whether in the intestinal tract or elsewhere in the body.

SIBO is like the new *Candida*, diagnosed frequently to explain all manner of symptoms and yet not truly understood. Although medical research and science are not yet aware, the bacterial overgrowth in SIBO is always strep. Unfortunately, doctors frequently offer antibiotics to treat SIBO. While that can get symptoms to subside in the moment, in many cases, it leads to worse bouts later—because this is a case of strep becoming immune to antibiotics and growing stronger.

Whether it's *Candida* or SIBO a practitioner has told you you're struggling with, celery juice is an excellent remedy. When you consume the juice, it directly enters the digestive tract, slowly traveling through the small intestinal tract and annihilating strep cells there. Here's an unexpected positive: celery juice will not hurt or hinder *Candida* as it goes. That's exactly what you want, since *Candida* is a beneficial fungus. In a way, celery juice is even smarter than conventional wisdom, because it knows not to destroy beneficial microorganisms in the gut the way that antibiotics do; celery juice knows to leave *Candida* alone and go after strep instead. *Candida*'s job is to gobble up harmful substances in your intestinal tract so strep cannot feed off them. Once you're destroying strep—the cause of SIBO—and cleansing those harmful substances that feed it by drinking celery juice, *Candida* will naturally go down to healthy levels. That is, *Candida* overgrowth is no longer needed when celery juice enters the system.

Whenever someone is dealing with SIBO, whether diagnosed or not, intestinal cramping and bloating usually occur. This comes from strep bacteria moving around the intestinal tract, creating little pockets of gas that can become uncomfortable. Celery juice addresses this by wiping out strep in the gut and assisting with digestion thanks to its digestive enzymes. (For more on bloating, turn back to page 40.)

Sore Throat and Strep Throat

People with strep throat can have strep bacteria within the lymphatic system and on the surface of the throat itself. Celery juice is so vital as both an offense and defense mechanism against strep throat because, as we covered, a person usually has multiple varieties of strep, many of them immune to antibiotics. Strep can't become immune to celery juice.

Have you heard of gargling salt water as a treatment for a sore throat? That doesn't deliver a fraction of the power that celery juice's sodium cluster salts deliver when a sip of celery juice flows down the throat. When consumed, celery juice helps pulverize strep bacteria rapidly on the surface of inflamed throat membranes. The cluster salts then bind onto the strep and carry the bacterial cells out of the body through elimination. A few hours later, celery juice's vitamin C and some of its remaining sodium cluster salts travel into the lymphatic system, hitting strep from behind. White blood cells—lymphocytes—use the cluster salts to seek out and destroy strep bacteria.

Now, some sore throats are viral, such as in the case of mononucleosis, commonly known as mono. Still, the majority of sore throats are caused by strep bacteria. Even when someone also has a virus, a sore throat can be strep-caused, since strep is a common cofactor to viruses. Often, a doctor will take a swab for a throat culture, and if it doesn't come back showing strep, they'll determine that it's not a strep-caused sore throat. What they don't realize is that just because strep isn't on the throat's surface doesn't mean it isn't hidden deep inside the lymphatic system, causing the symptom from the other side. Whether a sore throat is caused by strep on the throat's surface or beneath the surface and beyond detection, or by a virus, celery juice is a major ally. In the next chapter, you'll find an oral therapy to help especially with this symptom.

Urinary Tract Infections (UTIs), Bladder Infections, Bacterial Vaginosis (BV), and Yeast Infections

These conditions are all caused by the same problem: strep. Under the broad umbrella of UTIs, strep can reside in the bladder itself, causing a bladder infection, or it can reside in the ureters or urethra (or, as you saw earlier, in the kidneys). With BV, the discharge present, whether clear or discolored, comes from a chronic strep infection. And in the case of yeast infections, while yeast is present, it's not the cause of the infection; yeast overgrowth is only present because bacteria are present. While elevations of yeast can become cumbersome, they're not what's causing the pain or discomfort; strep is. This is often confused at the urologist's (and gynecologist's) office; the common practice is to identify the problem as yeast—mistakenly.

Celery juice travels into the kidneys and down through the rest of the urinary tract, with its powerful sodium cluster salts acting as a detergent along the way, attaching themselves to strep and assisting it out of the body through the urine. Reaching the reproductive system to take care of BV and yeast infections is a slightly more difficult journey. It's not quite as easy for it to reach the reproductive system through the bloodstream, so while some does reach it that way, celery juice also enters into the reproductive system through the lymphatic system in the groin. Once there, celery juice helps knock out strep so you can find relief.

TINNITUS

Ringing, Vibrating, or Buzzing in the Ears; Unexplained Hearing Loss

Long-term use of celery juice is most beneficial for tinnitus; ringing, vibrating, or buzzing in the ears; and unexplained hearing loss. When these issues are occurring with no obvious explanation—someone hasn't experienced decibel damage from working near machinery their whole life, playing music at high volumes, or similar strains to the eardrums—and it's a mystery to doctors, that means there's a virus present, one I cover extensively in *Medical Medium* and *Thyroid Healing*: the Epstein-Barr virus. When EBV releases neurotoxins into the bloodstream, they can find their way to the labyrinth of the inner ear. Here, they wreak havoc upon the nerves, causing mysterious inflammation. The virus itself may even enter the labyrinth, creating direct inflammation as well.

Yet again, we have celery juice's miraculous sodium cluster salts to thank for their antiviral power. Celery juice flushes viral neurotoxins out of the body, binding onto them and neutralizing them, while its cluster salts damage EBV and slow down its reproduction. These cluster salts also enter the inner ear's labyrinth and help restore nerve cells; nerve tissue takes trace minerals as protective fuel and nourishment to recover itself. While sometimes celery juice can get rid of tinnitus and similar symptoms quickly, for many, destroying EBV is a longer-term process, which is why drinking celery juice long term is your best course of action here. You'll further support the deep healing that needs to happen by taking additional steps that you'll find in Chapter 8 and the rest of the Medical Medium series.

THYROID CONDITIONS

Hypothyroidism; Hyperthyroidism; Graves' Disease; Hashimoto's Thyroiditis; Thyroid Nodules, Cysts, and Tumors; Goiters

These inflammatory thyroid conditions, which can range from mild inflammation to more extreme, are caused by the Epstein-Barr virus (EBV). The virus enters the thyroid, creating damage to the tissue there, and also takes up residence in other parts of the body, which is the true source of the symptoms that go along with thyroid problems. (More on that in *Thyroid Healing*.)

Celery juice's sodium cluster salts absorb into the thyroid, acting as an antiviral agent that strips the virus cells' outer membranes, which weakens the virus to the point that it either operates at diminished strength or dies off. Sodium cluster salts are extremely absorbable; they enter into thyroid tissue with ease, soaking deep into it so the thyroid can use these specialized mineral salts for rejuvenation and hormone development.

You know that eating celery sticks alone cannot have the same health effect as drinking celery juice. This is especially true when we're talking about thyroid healing. It would be easy to think that maybe celery juice's compounds absorb into the thyroid when passing through the throat. In truth, for celery juice's antiviral cluster salts to soak into the thyroid, they must be absorbed through the intestinal linings first and enter the bloodstream—that's how they travel to the thyroid.

An ailing thyroid usually means that it also contains a lot of viral debris such as dead viral casings, byproduct, and neurotoxins released by the virus. If this buildup is long term, it practically clogs thyroid tissue. Celery juice has such a cleansing, detoxifying effect when it finally reaches the thyroid. Its mineral salts bind onto the debris, helping remove it from the thyroid and improve the thyroid's condition. When thyroid nodules are present, celery juice also helps. Nodules are calcium prisons for EBV, and celery juice's sodium cluster salts help break down and dissolve these calcifications over time—at the same time they're going after the virus that created the nodules in the first place.

WEIGHT GAIN

When someone is gaining unwanted pounds, it means the liver has been collecting and storing an abundance of fat cells, creating a sluggish, stagnant, pre-fatty, or even undiagnosed fatty liver. That's right— weight gain is not a result of a slow metabolism. The *liver* is responsible for weight issues throughout all parts of the body. People who are dealing with weight issues are often also dealing with lymphatic

issues: lymphatic systems that are clogged up and harboring an abundance of fat cells because of that overloaded liver. When celery juice's chemical compounds enter the digestive system, absorb into the intestinal walls, go up the hepatic portal vein, and enter the liver, they start to revitalize liver cells. It's like a medicinal infusion for the liver.

Our liver is a filter that becomes clogged over time if we don't give it relief. Often, in addition to being clogged with fat cells, a sluggish, stagnant, or fatty liver is a sign that it's loaded with toxins that I call troublemakers. These can range from conventional detergents to colognes and perfumes to gasoline that you pump at the gas station to plug-in air fresheners to pesticides and herbicides to toxic heavy metals such as mercury, aluminum, and copper to old pharmaceuticals that have stayed trapped in your liver. As it gets clogged up, the liver loses its ability to function at its optimum level. Celery juice revitalizes the liver, helping to stimulate the organ while it removes toxins and poisons.

Celery juice's sodium cluster salts also bind onto viral debris in the liver—which is important, since everybody on Planet Earth is harboring pathogens inside their livers. Those pathogens range from the Epstein-Barr virus to shingles to HHV-6 and HHV-7 to cytomegalovirus to bacteria such as strep and *E. coli* and so much more. The liver becomes a nesting place for them when it's also filled with troublemakers because toxins and poisons actually feed pathogens. Celery juice's chemical compounds bind onto viral debris—viral byproduct and toxins—and help purge it from the liver. This strengthens and awakens the liver's ability to operate at its best and perform its over 2,000 chemical functions, most of them undiscovered. Celery juice also strips the membranes from pathogens in the liver, which weakens or kills them off. This is part of what allows celery juice to rejuvenate liver cell growth.

Finally, celery juice can break down and help dissolve fat cells that are stored inside the liver. It helps dislodge fat deposits there, breaking them down and breaking them free and cleansing these cells to remove fat storage from the liver. Plus, celery juice is loaded with vitamins and minerals that are separate from its sodium cluster salts, ones that help feed and strengthen the liver, making it less stagnant. Celery juice is a powerful weight-loss tool.

WEIGHT LOSS

Because celery juice is such a godsend to help shed unwanted pounds, people are sometimes concerned that they shouldn't try celery juice if they have the opposite problem—if they are underweight and *don't* want to lose any more weight. The truth is that you can still drink celery juice. It will actually help you, because celery juice assists in either circumstance, whether you're trying to gain or lose weight (or hold steady). It's a balancer.

Here's what's critical to know: Celery juice is not a meal replacement.

It's a medicine. Especially if you are underweight, you can't rely on celery juice as a calorie source. Don't skip a morning meal like a fruit smoothie that can provide healthy calories and replace it with a glass of celery juice. Have both: first, drink celery juice and then, after a minimum of 15 to 20 minutes and ideally a good 30 minutes, enjoy breakfast.

The reason celery juice helps with both weight gain and weight loss is that they both stem from a struggling liver. Unwanted, mystery weight loss is usually the result of a chronic, low-grade viral infection, such as EBV, inside the liver, setting off the body's alarm system, essentially creating an allergic reaction that prompts the adrenals to release consistently high levels of adrenaline. Basically, the adrenaline acts as an amphetamine. Often, mystery weight loss doesn't last forever, because eventually the liver becomes so tired, sluggish, and exhausted from fielding mass amounts of adrenaline that the situation flips, and people start gaining weight instead, even if it's ten years later.

Celery juice helps out with the viral situation that creates unwanted weight loss because its chemical compounds enter the liver's hepatic portal vein and break down viral cell membranes, which weakens and reduces the viral load, while celery juice's compounds also grab on to viral toxins—and such toxins as toxic heavy metals, pesticides, herbicides, and solvents that feed viruses—and pull them out of the liver. Celery juice's chemical compounds flow through the rest of the bloodstream, too, collecting and disengaging viral toxins floating throughout the body that are constantly setting off the mild, unseen allergic reactions that trigger the adrenals.

Often people with mystery weight loss have a higher heart rate, both when sleeping and awake. This is from leftover adrenaline surging through the body due to the allergic reaction to the viral load. Celery juice allows this to reverse over time so that weight can stabilize.

Remember: celery juice is not a calorie source. Do not expect to drink celery juice, not eat other foods, and start to gain weight. After you've given your morning celery juice 15 to 30 minutes to work through your system, you'll need to make sure you're getting healthy calories in your morning and the rest of your day. If they're part of the equation, celery juice can help you balance out. For insights on eating in a healthy manner, turn to Chapter 8, "More Healing Guidance."

MORE HEALING GEMS

If you didn't come across your symptom or condition in this chapter, remember: don't think celery juice cannot be beneficial for you. And if you did find your symptom or condition here, know that there's more to discover. Please look into other books in the Medical Medium series to find answers for your particular health issue. The series is packed with further information about what causes chronic health problems, along with protocols that incorporate celery juice so you can move forward with your healing. It's always great to check the series for additional gems that you may find very helpful for your individual health situation, since there wasn't nearly enough room here to give you all the details on every diagnosis.

After reading about these dozens of health issues and how celery juice can help, you're probably more motivated than ever to try celery juice or, if you've already tried it, to rededicate yourself to it. To make celery juice work best for you, you'll need to pay attention to a few key steps—and that's exactly what we're about to cover.

CHAPTER 4

How to Make Celery Juice Work for You

When we're talking about the benefits of celery juice, we need to be clear that we are talking about pure, straight, unadulterated celery *juice* and no other variation of it. We're not talking about a green juice blend that includes some celery. We're not talking about adding celery sticks to your smoothie. We're not talking about eating celery sticks. We're not talking about boiling celery in a broth. We're not talking about blending celery until it liquefies and then consuming it without straining.

While yes, celery itself is healthy—keep snacking on it and cooking with it and blending it—when it's prepared in these other ways, it doesn't offer the incomparable health benefits that drinking pure celery juice does. It's not even close.

The surprising reasons for this will become clearer as you read this chapter and beyond. For now, hold on to that key piece of wisdom: nothing equals the simple power of pure, fresh celery juice. You need to know this right up front so you won't be swayed by claims out there that any other preparation of celery is better for you.

(Not that you should panic if you don't have access to celery or for any other reason can't drink celery juice. There are alternatives available to you, and we'll get to those in Chapter 9.)

I don't want you to get lost in the maze of competing health claims. You could find yourself at a dead end with your health, following misleading theories that try to complicate what was never meant to be complicated. The knowledge in this book will ground you in the truth.

CELERY JUICE RECIPE
JUICER VERSION

Let's start with how to prepare celery juice properly. Making celery juice is beyond simple. If you have a juicer, here's all you'll need to do.

1 bunch celery

1. Trim about a quarter inch off the base of the celery bunch if desired to break apart the stalks.

2. Rinse the celery.

3. Run the celery through the juicer of your choice.

4. Strain the juice if desired to remove any grit or stray pieces of pulp.

5. Drink immediately, on an empty stomach, for best results.

6. Wait at least 15 to 30 minutes before consuming anything else.

(For reference, check out the photos on pages 90 and 91. You'll find more preparation tips starting on page 92.)

CELERY JUICE RECIPE

BLENDER VERSION

If you don't have access to a juicer, here's how you can make it in a blender instead.

1 bunch celery

1. Trim about a quarter inch off the base of the celery bunch if desired to break apart the stalks.

2. Rinse the celery.

3. Place the celery on a clean cutting board and chop into roughly one-inch pieces.

4. Place the chopped celery in a high-speed blender and blend until smooth. (Don't add water.) Use your blender's tamping tool if needed.

5. Strain the liquefied celery well. A nut milk bag is handy for this.

6. Drink immediately, on an empty stomach, for best results. Wait at least 15 to 30 minutes before consuming anything else.

JUICER VERSION

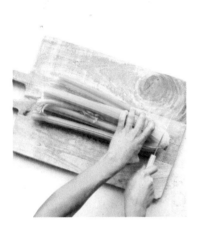

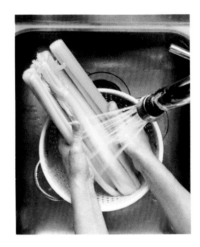

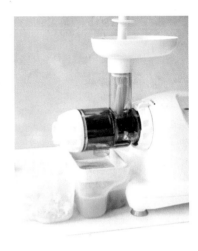

1. Trim about a quarter inch off the base of the celery bunch if desired to break apart the stalks.

2. Rinse the celery.

3. Run the celery through the juicer of your choice.

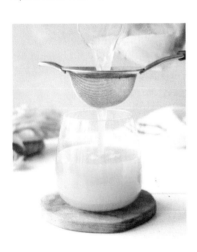

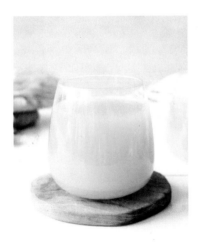

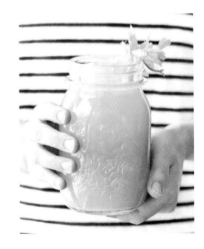

4. Strain the juice if desired to remove any grit or stray pieces of pulp.

5. Drink immediately, on an empty stomach, for best results.

6. Wait at least 15 to 30 minutes after drinking your celery juice before consuming anything else.

BLENDER VERSION

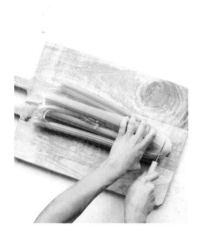

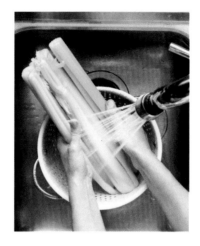

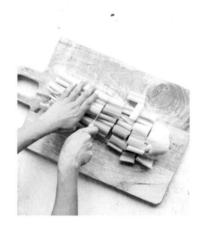

1. Trim about a quarter inch off the base of the celery bunch if desired to break apart the stalks.

2. Rinse the celery.

3. Place the celery on a clean cutting board and chop into roughly one-inch pieces.

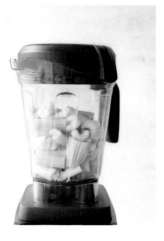

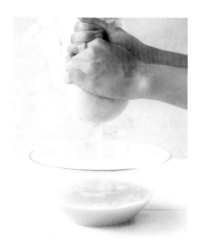

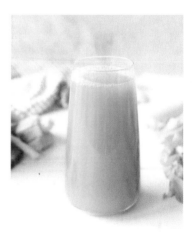

4. Place the chopped celery in a high-speed blender and blend until smooth. (Don't add water.) Use your blender's tamping tool if needed.

5. Strain the liquefied celery well. A nut milk bag is handy for this.

6. Drink immediately, on an empty stomach, for best results. Wait at least 15 to 30 minutes before consuming anything else.

PREPARATION TIPS

By the time you finish this book, you're going to be an expert on celery juice—and experts are always grounded in foundational knowledge. You've already picked up a lot of important information. Here are some more fundamentals for you.

Rinsing

When using store-bought celery, it's a good idea to give it a rinse before juicing. You can even turn your kitchen faucet to hot to rinse the celery, if it's chilled from the refrigerator and you don't want to drink cold celery juice. Washing it in hot water will reduce the celery's core temperature by at least 50 percent, meaning that you end up with more lukewarm celery juice. You'll learn quickly how to gauge what water temperature and length of rinsing time yield celery juice that you like.

You don't need to worry that washing your celery with hot tap water is going to cook your celery. You're not going to damage the celery's enzyme content or hinder it in any other way with this technique. It would take superheated water and a longer time in the water to do this.

When you're buying celery from a trusted local farmer or growing it in your own garden, then it's likely to be rich in what I call *elevated biotics*: undiscovered beneficial microorganisms on the surfaces of naturally grown fruits, vegetables, and herbs. In this case, it's usually best not to use hot water when rinsing the celery, unless the celery is caked with dirt, so you can avoid harming the elevated biotics. (You'll find more information on these incredible microorganisms and how they help us throughout the Medical Medium series.) Do feel free to give your local celery a rinse in more temperate water.

Conventional versus Organic

It is best to opt for organic whenever possible. If for any reason you can't get organic celery, don't worry. It's worth getting conventional celery rather than giving up on celery juice altogether. With conventional celery, take extra care by putting a drop of natural, fragrance-free dish soap on each stalk and then washing with it and rinsing well.

Taste

Everyone's first taste of celery juice is unique. Some people aren't wild about it at first and come to love it over time. Others find it appealing from the get-go. So much of this depends on how many toxins are in the system when people first try celery juice. If somebody is dealing with a lot of toxins, celery juice can be a shock to the system. As it binds onto troublemakers and flushes them out of the liver, our senses can actually detect them—our taste buds and sense of smell can be affected. Toxins have a way of turning deliciousness into sourness or other unpleasant flavors. This will pass. Some people who don't like celery juice on the first day love it by the end of the week. Some people may need six months of drinking it to really appreciate and crave it. People have a range of toxic, overburdened bodies and livers, so it all depends. There's a trend of adding squeezed lemon to celery juice to alter the taste. By doing this, you'll disable celery juice's healing powers. You'll get more benefits from drinking a lower quantity of pure celery juice than you will from drinking a high quantity of celery juice that has lemon added. For those who need help adjusting to the juice's flavor, a smaller glass is better than a large one that has a squeeze of lemon.

One person's experience of celery juice can change from day to day—even if it's all from the same store, same farm, same batch, same case, and stocked on the same shelf on the same day. Part of that could be that you're detoxing your dinner from the night before, or it could be that you drank some coffee last night or brushed your teeth right before drinking your celery juice.

The flavor and color of celery juice can change from batch to batch, too. Over time, you're likely to notice that you come home from the store with different types of celery that result in different types of celery juice. Some weeks, it's greener. Some weeks, it has more leaves. Some weeks, it's darker and more spindly; these wispier stalks tend to yield juice that's a little more bitter and therefore maybe a little harder to get down. Some weeks, you'll find large, crisp stalks that provide lots of juice and a salty flavor with maybe even a hint of sweetness. Some weeks, you can barely taste the sodium content, even though the beneficial sodium cluster salts are still there. It all varies depending on what farm grew it with what

type of seed with what type of soil amendments with what irrigation at what time of year in what type of weather conditions.

Try not to be turned off when you get a less palatable, less juicy batch of celery; these bunches can actually be a little more medicinal. Also don't worry if you find lighter celery, almost translucent toward the bottom—don't pass on this. It's okay if it was wrapped during growing in a blanching process. Lighter celery is often more palatable, which means you can get more in you, so there is a plus side to it. Even with less chlorophyll, this celery will still provide other phytochemical compounds that help you heal. Further, celery juice's chlorophyll is more powerful than the chlorophyll from any other source, because it's bonded to the sodium cluster salts, plant hormones, and vitamin C that only celery possesses. This means that *any* chlorophyll you get in your celery juice, even if it's a small amount, will be more potent than what you can get anywhere else.

You'll see it all as you learn your way around the land of celery. Whatever celery you find, it will still provide the sodium cluster salts that you've read so much about and all of celery juice's other valuable nutritional components. Whatever celery it is—as long as it's not celery root—it will make celery juice that will help you heal.

Celery Leaves

People often ask about the leaves of celery—if they're good for you and whether you should juice them. The answer is that celery leaves are extremely medicinal.

They're loaded with minerals and other nutrients and even beneficial plant hormones. Still, that doesn't mean you have to use them. The flavor of celery leaves can be very bitter, so if the taste of your celery juice turns you off, try trimming the leaves, either partly or all the way, before juicing and see if that makes the juice more palatable.

Store-bought celery tends to have only so many leaves left on it. Celery that you grow yourself or that you buy from a farmers' market often has an abundance of leaves. When using local or homegrown celery, I prefer that you trim some of the leaves back and make sure that the majority of what you're juicing is celery stalk. Too many celery leaves can give juice an astringency that makes it less enjoyable, so you may not want to drink as much of it. Too many leaves can also lead to more rapid detox, again making the overall experience of celery juice less enjoyable and making it less likely that you'll keep going with it. Since store-bought celery usually doesn't have as many leaves, your choice whether or not to juice them really only depends on your own taste and preference.

Whether celery leaves register as bitter for you depends in part on whether you've acquired a taste for bitter greens in your diet. If you have had bitter greens on salads for years, celery leaves may seem no different from any other herb. The reason celery leaves are bitter is because of the alkaloids they contain. These phytochemical compounds are very strong to our taste buds; they can be a little intense. That's perfectly normal and natural. They are not toxic alkaloids. While some alkaloids in other plants can be toxic in nature, this is not a concern with celery. Celery's alkaloids are medicinal and very detoxifying. They help alkalize the body and reduce acids that are toxic in nature and that reside in our organs and elsewhere internally. In particular, celery leaves' alkaloids help purge toxins from our livers.

By the way, when I'm making celery juice, I like to chop about a half an inch off the tips of the celery bunch (the leaf end) and about a quarter inch off the base (the root end) before I start juicing. This has nothing to do with the leaves themselves. Rather, you'll usually see that the celery has been cut on each end before. I trim it further because I don't know what tool was used to cut the celery—whether it was clean, dirty, used near livestock, done by machine or hand, or whether there was grease on it. You don't have to do this if you prefer to use every bit of your celery for juice. Chances are all is fine, and a clean tool was used to harvest your celery. This is solely a personal decision I've made.

Juicers

Any juicer that will juice celery is going to serve you. That celery juice is going to be beneficial to you. Rest easy with that knowledge. If you already own a juicer, it's the right juicer. Please continue using it.

If you're in the market for a juicer, either because you don't own one yet or you'd like to upgrade, a masticating juicer is ideal. It will preserve and extract the most nutrition from the celery and make the least noise. Masticating juicers also get the most juice out of your celery, meaning more juice per bunch of celery—as well as less foam and pulp.

All that said, a centrifugal juicer is okay if that's what works for your life. This type tends to be faster, so if what's standing between you and celery juice is the time it takes to make it, a centrifugal juicer may solve that problem. Look for one that keeps the fruits and vegetables cool as it juices them, rather than heating them up the way some high-speed juicers can.

If all you have right now is a high-speed blender or food processor, you'll probably find yourself wanting to get a juicer someday. The blending method tends to yield less juice than using a juicer, and the extra step of straining the blended celery can get old after a while. Remember, though: whatever machine you're using right now to make celery juice, it's a good machine. Don't feel discouraged if you're not using the highest-end masticating juicer. You're still making great juice that will benefit your body in untold ways.

Juice Bars

It's fine to get your fresh celery juice from a juice bar, juice store, café, or the juice counter of a natural foods store rather than making it yourself.

If it's cold-pressed celery juice, that's great. Not that I want anyone to become fixated on going out and buying cold-pressed juice, thinking that's the only way to go. Cold-pressed celery juice is not the only way to get its nutrients. Purchasing celery

juice made with a centrifugal juicer is good, too. And juicing celery at home with a good, old-fashioned masticating juicer is just as beneficial as fancy cold-pressed juice from a store. *Any* type of juicer you have at home can create celery juice that's nutritious.

If you still prefer to go out and buy your celery juice, there are a couple of considerations to take into account.

First, ask how they prepare the celery. Some places will put a drop of chlorine or bleach in with the water when they're washing produce before juicing. You don't want this.

Second, if the celery juice you're buying is pre-bottled, check the label carefully to make sure it doesn't say "HPP" anywhere. Sometimes it's in small print or there's a little symbol for it. Even if it doesn't list it, ask the clerk to make sure it isn't HPP. If it is, please consider picking another juice source that makes celery juice fresh on location. You do not want HPP celery juice.

HPP stands for *high-pressure pasteurization*, and it means that rather than being freshly cold-pressed, bottled, and put on the shelf for you that day, the juice was delivered from a manufacturing plant. The pasteurization process of HPP doesn't require heat, and this can lead to the illusion that it's raw. Quite the contrary. Juice that's been put through HPP has been denatured. Its cell structures have changed shape and form through this new process that hasn't been time tested. Regular pasteurization is a heating process that's shown its safety over the course of hundreds of years. Not that you want regularly pasteurized celery juice, either—you want it fresh and raw. Assuming that HPP means it's raw juice is a mistaken assumption, though. In theory, it's raw. In reality, it's been hindered and compromised to sustain shelf life. The reason to be wary of HPP is that it's not going to bring you the health benefits of celery juice. I can see many people picking up HPP celery juice, trying it for a while, and then giving up because their symptoms and conditions haven't improved. Don't let that be you.

HPP for other fruit and vegetable juices can still provide nutrients, so if you're used to consuming those HPP juices and you want to continue, you will get some benefits. Celery, on the other hand, is an herb. Because of this, HPP will cause the loss of multiple miraculous benefits that it has to offer, including some of its most important ones. When it comes to herbal medicines such as celery juice, if you've lost even one of its benefits, you've lost an opportunity to heal.

Storing Celery

If you're regularly making your own celery juice, you may want to see if you can buy celery by the case from your local grocer. Ask the produce department if they have a case to spare or if they can add a case to their next order. You'll often receive a discount, plus, you're likely to end up with fresher celery that will last longer at home. It will also save you from running out as often.

Celery itself will usually keep in the fridge for a week. I've seen celery hold out, staying green and crisp, for up to two weeks if it was a really strong, fresh batch at the start. One way to determine your celery's viability is color. Try to use it up before it starts to turn yellow or brown and loses its green color. If there's ever a time when your busy life takes over and celery that you've purchased turns before you've gotten a chance to use it, don't lose heart at having to throw it away. Don't let that turn you off celery juice. Please buy yourself some new celery and try again.

If you're buying celery and planning to use it up quickly, you should be fine storing it any way you'd like in the fridge. After a few days, celery sitting uncovered on the shelf is likely to dry out and go floppy. To prevent this, the crisper drawers of a refrigerator are a great place to store it. Sometimes celery comes in plastic sleeves, or you've put it in produce bags at the store. In that case, it should keep fine without the crisper. If you've bought a case of celery and it didn't come in plastic sleeves, grab some produce bags from the roll at the store—the produce department will likely be happy to send you home with them, since they just sold you an entire case.

Storing Celery Juice

If you're not going to be able to drink your full batch of celery juice right away, the best way to store it is in a glass jar, with a sealed lid, in the fridge. Freshly juiced celery retains its healing benefits for about 24 hours. It will technically keep for about three days in the fridge—although it won't be of much help to you after the first day. Celery juice loses potency by the hour, so drinking it more than 24 hours after it's made is far from ideal.

You can freeze celery juice, although that's not ideal, either. If it's your only option, though, then go ahead and freeze it—I'd recommend in ice cube trays for ease of use—and when you're ready, take it out and drink it as soon as it's thawed. Don't add water to the celery juice cubes, though, and don't thaw the frozen celery juice cubes in water. That will interfere with its benefits.

I wouldn't freeze celery itself. Freezing stalks, defrosting them, and juicing them will not lead to a good outcome. Even though it seems comparable to freezing the juice, it's not. When you juiced the celery fresh, you extracted its life force. If you were to freeze the celery, you would end up juicing a lifeless stalk later.

You definitely don't want to boil your celery or celery juice—unless, that is, you're intentionally making a broth. You can go ahead and put celery in your soups and stews; celery in your diet on a regular basis is helpful for a number of conditions. Still, when you boil celery, you're destroying the enzymes and denaturing some of its nutrients. It won't be the hard-hitting, healing medicinal that you need celery juice to be. It won't help you move the needle forward. That's the job of freshly juiced celery.

WHY 16 OUNCES?

The ideal amount of celery juice for most adults is a minimum of 16 ounces per day. Not that you have to or necessarily want to start with 16 ounces the first time you try it. Feel free to work your way up, starting with 4 or 8 ounces if you're sensitive and from there increasing it a little every day as you get used to it.

Once you're ready, it is a good idea to commit to those 16 ounces as a minimum. Why? Because most people have more than a few health obstacles to overcome. The celery juice must travel quite a distance on its journey. Its first obstacle is often in the mouth, with bacteria or leftover toothpaste, mouthwash, or mouth rinse. (Make sure to thoroughly rinse your mouth with fresh water after brushing your teeth and before drinking celery juice to get rid of any toothpaste, mouthwash, or mouth rinse residue. Even better, wait to brush your teeth until after you've had your morning celery juice.)

Then there's the esophagus, where the celery juice encounters additional bacteria plus deposits of ammonia and unproductive, detrimental acids. Next it reaches a hurdle at the bottom of the stomach pouch, just before the duodenum (the entrance to the small intestine). There's a little ledge right before the duodenum, and depending on someone's age, that alone can be filled with decades—sometimes 30 to 40 years' worth—of debris that has gummed up and weighed down that little cliff. This debris could be from proteins, fats, preservatives, solidified ammonia, acids, and more, all of it corroding and formed into a sludgy deposit. Celery juice's sodium cluster salts start eating away at this old pile of toxic sludge, slowly dissolving it over time.

So first the celery juice has to get through those obstacles. Then, as the celery juice is moving through the duodenum, it's usually met with a barrage of *H. pylori*, *Streptococcus*, and other varieties of bacteria—because most people live with undiagnosed cases of these bacteria. Celery juice has to fight to sustain itself and stay active in this battle, which is doubly hard since it was already defused from dealing with toothbrushing residues and bacteria in the mouth; ammonia, acid, and more bacteria in the esophagus; and debris as it left the stomach.

As it continues through the duodenum, celery juice is bombarded with acids, since most everybody's pH is "off" internally in this day and age. It's not like we're automatically alkaline. Sure, if someone's healthy, their pH will be pretty balanced, and celery juice won't have to do much work in this respect. Most people are filled with bacteria, though, and that's a big acid producer. Unproductive diets and punishing stress levels are acid producers, too. As soon as we take our first sip, celery juice starts altering the internal pH of the body, beginning with the mouth and continuing down the digestive tract. It's almost like an explosion as celery juice tries to turn the tide of high acidity, and that's yet one more source that defuses it in its travels through our system.

Sound like a lot for celery juice to encounter and keep up its strength? There's more. Just a few inches farther in the small intestinal tract, celery juice encounters a slick of mucus. It's there in young and old alike—a layer of bottom feeders like strep and *E. coli* and other unproductive bacteria, usually along with two to three unproductive funguses, all of them just waiting

for protein from eggs or supplemental collagen that we consume, or lactose from milk, cheese, butter, or other dairy, so the bugs can feed on them. When celery juice instead hits this pathway of pathogens, it's yet one more area of battle.

Plus, there are rancid fats that have hardened and caked along the intestinal wall linings from years of high-fat foods, whether from healthy or unhealthy fat sources, as well as rotting protein that has formed into little balls of debris and created pockets in the intestinal tract that guard more bacteria and funguses. Addressing all of this is yet one more series of obstacles for celery juice during its travels.

That's not even everything; it only describes the major hurdles that celery juice encounters so far. Then add in excess adrenaline—say, if you ate on the run or under stress, with tension in your gut, or if you ate too much fat with your meal the night before without realizing it, any of which prompts the adrenals to release a burst of adrenaline. When this excess adrenaline enters the intestinal tract, it's a scorcher. It saturates cells all through the body, so if you were under intense stress or encountered another adrenal trigger the day before, when you wake up the next day, the adrenaline is still sitting in the intestinal tract. Celery juice works on neutralizing this adrenaline: yet one more battle. While celery juice will try to handle it, that's a tall order considering everything else it went through as it traveled along through the gut.

A high-fat dinner does more than trigger adrenaline. Fats left over from dinner linger in the gut, from the stomach to the small intestinal tract to the colon, like an oil slick, and celery juice is up against those, too. High levels of these fats soak up celery juice's healing compounds, using up sodium cluster salts, since they must go to work dispersing those fats and cleaning them out of the digestive tract. This means that if someone has an extra heavy dinner, maybe with something fried for the main course followed by dessert, celery juice will need to work extra hard the next morning, and that will diminish some of its healing power as it continues on the obstacle course.

The digestive system was only the beginning. The majority of the world is also dealing with stagnant, sluggish livers, and here's the critical part: enough celery juice has to make it to the colon with its potency intact to be absorbed into the bloodstream so celery juice's compounds can travel through the hepatic portal vein into the liver and then into the gallbladder—to help you heal. Regardless of what you're dealing with in life, a healthier liver means a greater chance of healing any variety of symptom or condition you're up against. Sixteen ounces is the magic number to do this for the majority of adults. (More soon on amounts for children.)

Once celery juice does get to the liver, it encounters another set of hurdles. For one, most people's livers are toxic with poisons, pesticides, herbicides, plastics and other petrochemicals, solvents, pathogens such as viruses and bacteria, and many more troublemakers. All of this strains the liver's bile production. When celery juice's compounds enter the bile production area, if they're still potent enough, they will improve the strength of the bile that the liver sends to the gallbladder. This celery juice–bolstered bile then starts dismantling and dispersing sludge in the gallbladder while also breaking down and dissolving gallstones. If you've been drinking large enough quantities of celery juice for long enough to get your system clean and healthy, celery juice's compounds will then leave the gallbladder with the bile as it's released into the intestinal tract. This is part of celery juice's responsibility: to come full circle.

Not all of celery juice's healing components that make it to the liver get directed to the bile. Some leave the liver through the bloodstream, heading up to the heart and brain, although their healing abilities by this point are pretty minimal if someone has a sluggish or stagnant liver, which most people do. It takes time for someone to clean up the liver to the point that celery juice's components still hold benefits as they exit this way.

That's okay, though, because celery juice has another way of getting its potent components to the bloodstream. Back when celery juice was first in the digestive tract, only some of it—roughly half—traveled to the liver in the first place. It divided itself on the obstacle course. While traveling through the stomach and the first 36 inches of the small intestine, the other half of celery juice's chemical compounds absorbed into the digestive tract walls and entered the bloodstream directly without going to the liver first. Traveling through the blood is its own set of hurdles. How much fat is in the blood? (Fats interfere with celery juice's travel distance.) How many toxins are in the blood? How many toxic heavy metals are inside various organs such as the brain? Speaking of the brain, how many neurotransmitter chemical issues are occurring there? All of this defuses and weakens any strength that celery juice has left. If neurotransmitter chemicals in the brain are diminished, celery juice's compounds get used up in instantly replacing them, making this their final destination, in a way. If heavy metals need to be dislodged, celery juice's sodium cluster salts get consumed with helping them out of the body.

Given the gargantuan scope of celery juice's job, you can see why you'd want to drink enough of it to get that job done. The next time someone is quizzing you about why you drink this particular amount of celery juice, well, it's up to you. You could give them the play-by-play of its travels through the digestive tract and beyond (in which case you probably want to make sure they aren't eating!). You could give them the condensed version: celery juice has huge responsibilities and an obstacle course to overcome as it travels through your body and works on healing it. Or you could hand them this book. Whichever you choose, now *you* know, and that's critical, because connecting to the "whys" of celery juice makes it all the more powerful.

Larger Quantities

It's okay to do more than 16 ounces of celery juice. Thirty-two ounces of celery juice a day is really helpful for people who are suffering from autoimmune disease and other chronic illness, sometimes taken as 16 ounces in the morning and 16 ounces in the afternoon or evening. Also, athletes can benefit and improve their game or performance if they increase to 32 ounces a day or even more. It's okay for people to go up to 64 ounces of celery juice daily, although in that case, it takes some adjustment—some people may experience the frequent urge to use the bathroom because they're cleansing and detoxing more.

What you don't want to do is wake up one day and say, "I've never had celery juice before. Let me start with sixty-four ounces." Celery juice is going to cause some cleansing and purging in your system as its sodium cluster salts break down and kill off pathogens and escort the pathogens' toxic waste matter out of the body and bloodstream through the skin, kidneys (via urination), and intestinal tract (via defecation). Especially if you're sensitive or dealing with a lot of toxins in your system, or if you live with a virus such as Epstein-Barr (causing, for example, fibromyalgia, MS, lupus, Hashimoto's, PCOS, ME/CFS, RA, and symptoms such as tingles, numbness, aches, pains, and fatigue) or live with bacteria such as strep (causing a condition such as SIBO, sinus infections, UTIs, sties, ear infections, and sore throats), you're likely to experience that cleansing and purging. I recommend that first-timers start with 16 ounces or less and graduate to higher quantities over time if it feels right. You could start with 4 ounces, and then every single day, a little at a time, keep graduating until you reach 16 ounces.

If you want to do more, then you can work your way up to 32 ounces per day. If you want to do even more, don't go straight to 64 ounces from there. Go to 40 ounces daily first and then graduate to 64 to ease your body into larger volumes of this medicinal. If you're feeling extreme, you can do a little more than 64 ounces—you can go up to 80 ounces—although you should cap it there. You don't want to do more than 80 ounces in a 24-hour period.

Amounts for Children

Babies and children don't have the multitude of obstacles in their guts for celery juice to traverse, so they don't need as much celery juice. Here's a guide to amounts for young ones. These are recommended daily minimums. It can be less if that feels right for your child, or more. You don't need to worry that going over these minimums is harmful.

Age	Amount
6 months old	1 ounce or more
1 year old	2 ounces or more
18 months old	3 ounces or more
2 years old	4 ounces or more
3 years old	5 ounces or more
4 to 6 years old	6 to 7 ounces or more
7 to 10 years old	8 to 10 ounces or more
11 years old and up	12 to 16 ounces

Skinny Stalks with More Leaves

You may live in an area or country where the only celery available has small, dark, skinny stalks and tons of leaves, and one whole bunch yields just a few ounces of juice. It's okay in this circumstance if you can only get a small glass of celery juice in yourself. Even though you won't get the complete benefits of 16 or more ounces of milder celery juice, you will get the next best thing. As I mentioned in "Preparation Tips," celery's chlorophyll is uniquely beneficial, bonded to celery's sodium cluster salts, plant hormones, and vitamin C. The richness and intensity of the chlorophyll you'll get from this deep green celery will in part compensate for the lower quantity of juice, and it will still help with healing different aspects of your body. I highly recommend juicing whatever celery you can access rather than giving up altogether because you can only get small dosages. After all, it's still celery—its juice will still move you forward. You can also help compensate by immersing yourself in other Medical Medium information to ensure you're moving forward on all levels.

WHY PURE CELERY JUICE ON AN EMPTY STOMACH?

To get the benefits of celery juice that we're looking at throughout this book, it's important to drink celery juice on an empty stomach. That's vital to remember. Otherwise—if, say, you drank your celery juice right along with your breakfast or had it with an afternoon snack—you would miss out on its full healing power. It would still be beneficial, just not to anywhere near the degree it's meant to be.

The same diminished power goes for drinking a juice blend. If you go to the store and see a fresh juice that lists spinach, beets, ginger, lemon, and celery—and highlights celery on the label as if that makes it celery juice—be a savvy consumer. Celery juice is a one-ingredient drink. Even a juice blend of celery plus one other ingredient—say, celery-apple juice or celery-cucumber juice or celery-lemon juice—throws off the benefits that you want when you first get up for the day. If you like other juice blends, that's great; they're good for you. Save them for later in the day. For your special 16-ounce celery juice on an empty stomach, make it celery only.

The reasons for this are very specific. One has to do with celery's undiscovered subgroup of sodium; that is, the sodium cluster salts you read about in Chapter 2 and then throughout Chapter 3, mentioned over and over again for their unique ability to defend you and help you say good-bye to symptoms and conditions. Sodium cluster salts are some of the most powerful components of celery juice—they're behind so many of the dramatic transformations in the health of those who start drinking it—and they need to be consumed on an empty stomach in order to do their job right. Not that you need to panic if there's a day when you need to have breakfast first and drink your celery juice later. In that case, refer to "Timing Tips" in a few pages.

Benefits to the Brain

The brain is usually a difficult place to get anything into due to the blood-brain barrier. Sodium cluster salts, on the other hand, can reach the brain and benefit it as the ultimate electrolytes because their ability to cross the blood-brain barrier is unmatched. We're talking natural electrolytes, not manufactured, and those in celery juice can travel with higher velocity and reach than any other food-based electrolyte or manufactured drink or supplement. For all of this to work, though, celery juice needs to be on its own, and it does need to be celery *juice*. Eating celery won't deliver enough of the sodium cluster salts to your system to even travel to the brain. And if you mix celery with other ingredients, you get a similar problem: those additional fruits or vegetables or other add-ins dilute the celery juice, meaning you don't get enough of it or its sodium cluster salts.

Whether you're eating celery or blending it or tossing in an extra like a collagen supplement to your juice, those additional components interrupt sodium cluster salts' ability to benefit you. Fiber, fat, and protein particularly get in the way. (More on fiber in a few pages.) They stop sodium cluster salts from being able to bind onto important nutrients such as other minerals and amino acids, and they prevent the cluster salts from traveling and delivering those nutrients to the brain. Further, as you'll read about in "Timing Tips" in this chapter, as well as in Chapter 5, "The Celery Juice Cleanse," I recommend enjoying your celery juice apart from any fats, because fats trigger your liver to release bile to help digest them, and too much bile dilutes the sodium cluster salts, too.

If you add celery to your smoothie, the cluster salts won't get to your brain. If you blend up whole celery and drink it with the fiber still in it, the cluster salts won't get to your brain. If you eat celery sticks instead of juicing them, drink celery juice when your stomach is full of other food, put celery in with other ingredients in a green juice, or add collagen, activated charcoal, apple cider vinegar, or any other newly thought-of misguided idea to your celery juice, the cluster salts won't get to your brain. They'll get too bogged down.

Pathogen Protection

All of that *plus* another job of sodium cluster salts is to kill off pathogens. Only pure celery juice on an empty stomach allows cluster salts the direct contact with viruses, bacteria, and funguses they need for their fast-killing action. The minute you mix celery juice with juiced apples, spinach, or kale, or with protein powder, pea protein, collagen, nutritional yeast, or any other add-in, you lose this benefit completely.

Whatever you combine celery juice with, whether bad or good, prevents the sodium cluster salts from making direct contact with yeast, mold, food-borne toxins, *Streptococcus*, *Staphylococcus*, *E. coli*, *H. pylori*, HPV, EBV, and other toxic microbes. You lose the hardcore pathogen smack-down benefit.

If you follow a belief system that fresh, raw fruit and vegetable juices are too cold for the body or cause dampness, and someone recommends that you add ginger, turmeric, or cayenne to your celery juice to warm it up, know this: there's nothing wrong with adding these spices to your celery juice—if you're not concerned with getting the full spectrum of celery juice's benefits. To get everything out of celery juice, though, it needs to be pure, straight, and unadulterated. If you want ginger, turmeric, or cayenne, have them with something else, maybe even in another vegetable juice later in the day. Plain and simple fresh celery juice, believe it or not, is actually the best remedy for what Eastern medicine identifies as heat and dampness issues in the body, because it restores and revitalizes the liver, the very source of the problem.

Gut Glory

Diluting celery juice with any other ingredients also causes you to miss out on its benefits to your gut. That's a shame, both because celery juice has such restorative powers for digestion and because a well-functioning gut leads to celery juice being absorbed and assimilated better so it can assist the rest of the body. Celery juice's sodium cluster salts and digestive enzymes together can break up and dispel mucus and toxic acid in the digestive tract as well as old fats that have become caked on the walls of the small intestine and colon. Everyone has these fats clinging to their digestive tract walls. They aren't just fats

from fried oils, hydrogenated oils, grease, or saturated fat sources. Buildup can also occur from fat sources that are considered to be the healthiest around—including nuts, seeds, avocados, and high-quality oils—if they're being eaten day in and day out from morning until night. Most people would be shocked to learn the amount of fat they really consume and what that's doing to their body. (By the way, remember those digestive enzymes from Chapter 2? They'll work only if celery juice is by itself when it enters the small intestine.)

Taken on an empty stomach, pure celery juice also has an ignition power that allows it to be absorbed into your intestinal walls and bloodstream. This is critical, as it's what allows celery juice's components to work their way through your brain and body and deliver their healing power. We're dealing with so much. When celery juice enters our bodies, it has a lot of fish to fry. Getting it through this vital step—being absorbed into the bloodstream—makes it possible for sodium cluster salts to get where they need to go so they can benefit the brain, kill off bugs, dissolve hardened fats from artery linings, help cleanse the liver, and more. Tampering with celery juice's purity impedes these intended hard-hitting actions.

I understand. It's human nature to want to tamper with something so pure. Everyone has an inner alchemist, an inner mixologist. We like to tinker, put things into other things in the hopes of making better things. That's one reason why celery juice has been disregarded as a healing mechanism. We're not comfortable if something is already in its highest form and our human ingenuity can't improve upon it. It's why recipes are so popular instead of eating simply, in mono form, one food at a time. When we eat, we want to incorporate more than one ingredient. When we drink, we itch to mix and blend. Our mind-set is "What's next?" It's difficult to compute that there is no next and that celery juice holds a particular value and merit that's above all this. Instead, we decide celery juice must not be good enough on its own to do anything for anyone. Even with all the stories of people's healing from pure celery juice, so many observers can't stop themselves from diluting it with water or adding ice cubes or keeping the pulp in or adding a shot of this or a shot of that, inadvertently messing it up. When you get the bug to improve upon celery juice, know this: adhering to the guidelines of pure celery juice on an empty stomach is the secret that eludes those who tamper with it. You don't need to worry that it's too plain or simplistic. It already is the better thing. *You've already performed the alchemy by turning celery into celery juice.* You've already transformed it into gold.

THE FIBER QUESTION

People frequently wonder why juicing celery is the key, rather than eating it or blending it and then drinking it unstrained. Isn't it better to get celery's fiber and benefit from the whole food? This is an excellent question. You've already discovered part of the answer, which is that the fiber blocks celery's sodium cluster salts from doing all their intended jobs.

Here's what else you need to know: celery is an herb, and celery juice is a medicine that you make from it. When you make herbal tea, you're not concerned with consuming the whole herb. You don't hear that you're missing out because you don't chew all the leaves from your tea bag. You're concerned with extracting the herb's medicine. That's how it is with celery. In this case, instead of pouring hot water over it the way you do with tea, you're running it through a juicer to extract and unlock all its potent offerings.

That whole foods are automatically better—that blending is better than juicing because it leaves the fiber intact—is a belief system. It's a theory. Celery juice isn't about belief systems or theories. It's bigger. This is a miracle herbal medicine. People are so used to ignoring or disregarding celery that they don't connect to this. It's not understood that in order to make celery work for us on the level we need, we have no choice other than to extract it as juice. When someone lives by a belief system powered by professionals who posit that it's better to leave the pulp or fiber with celery, it's really telling you that they're unaware of celery juice's role, what it really is, and how uniquely different it is separated from its fiber. This isn't your standard vegetable juice. It's herbal medicine. Trendy belief systems have no place when it comes to healing from chronic conditions. If someone claims that the fiber must stay intact, it shows they're misinformed about the power of celery juice. It shows that they're lost and they don't know the history of what celery juice has done for thousands and thousands of people through the decades.

Fiber is great. Keep eating fiber! If you're worried about getting more fiber in your diet, go ahead and add more fibrous plant foods to your day. Even eat some celery sticks, if you want—later on, after you've had your celery juice. If you're already eating a lot of plant foods and not many processed foods, chances are you're already getting plenty of fiber. As great as fiber is, and as great as the fiber in celery is, you still don't want it in your celery juice. If you decide to blend up celery without straining the pulp, the fiber will actually block some of celery juice's benefits, plus, it will bulk up the liquid and keep you from drinking enough celery juice to tap into its healing power.

If, once you've juiced your celery, you seem to have a little fine pulp or grit floating in it and you don't like this, you're welcome to strain it with a fine mesh strainer, colander, or nut milk bag. Don't worry about it, though, unless you have a hypersensitive intestinal tract. Wondering if that's you? If you're afraid of raw vegetables and salads because you find them irritating to the gut, that probably means you have a hypersensitive intestinal tract. In that case, go ahead and strain your celery juice. By doing this, you ensure that you can drink larger quantities of celery juice.

For others, it's a matter of personal preference. When you've used a proper juicer, if you aren't hypersensitive, you can leave these few tiny, fibrous pieces in the juice— they're okay to consume and won't interfere with celery juice's potency, since the bulk of the pulp has been removed. Or if you'd like, go ahead and strain it. The straining step *is* critical for folks who are blending their celery in a high-speed blender or food processor, though. Drinking a shred or two of celery pulp in celery you've juiced in a juicer is far different from drinking unstrained, blended celery and thinking that you're getting the same benefits.

As for what to do with the leftover pulp from juicing, my only recommendation is to use it as compost for your garden.

TIMING TIPS

The ideal approach is to drink your celery juice in the morning, before you consume anything else besides water. (If you work a night shift, then have your celery juice whenever you get up, whether in the afternoon or evening.) Once you've finished your celery juice, wait at least 15 to 20 minutes, and ideally 30 minutes, before eating or drinking anything else.

If you do drink plain water or lemon or lime water before your celery juice, that's a great option as long as you space out the water and the celery juice. Water upon waking gives your liver a gentle flush and provides hydration to all your cells before you dive in to the medicine chest that is celery juice. (Drinking lemon water first thing in the morning in order to cleanse the liver is a tip that originated from my lectures decades ago, back when I was traveling around talking about celery juice and more. It's advice that caught on more easily than celery juice, because people were less skeptical of lemons and water—plus, it offered that sense of alchemy we crave.) Make sure to wait—at least 15 to 20 minutes if you're in a hurry and ideally 30 minutes—after finishing your water before drinking your celery juice. If you'd like to drink water *after* your celery juice, then the same spacing guideline applies: after finishing your celery juice, wait at least 15 to 20 minutes and ideally 30 minutes before drinking your water.

Now, what if you are not in a position to drink celery juice on an empty stomach in the morning, when it is most beneficial? Don't let that stop you from having it at all. To begin with, if it's because you won't have time when you get up, consider juicing your celery the night before and storing it in an airtight jar in the fridge for when you get up.

If that's not an option, and you can't get to celery juice until after breakfast, or if you want to have a second serving in the afternoon, celery juice still can and will be helpful taken at these other times of day. You just need to be mindful of food in your system getting in the way of celery juice's job and purpose and what it's trying to do. Timing your celery juice depends on what you've been eating. If you last had a meal that was high in fat and protein, meaning that it contained ingredients like chicken, beef, eggs, cheese, avocado, nuts, seeds, peanut butter, other nut or seed butters, or oils, it's best to wait a minimum of two hours and ideally three hours before having your celery juice. If you last ate something lighter, such as fresh fruit, oatmeal, or salad

(that wasn't loaded with high-fat options like olives, anchovies, bacon, tuna, nut butter, seeds, or oil-based dressing), then you can drink your celery juice 30 to 60 minutes after eating. Either way, after you've had your celery juice, wait a minimum of 15 to 30 minutes until you eat or drink anything else.

By the way, if you ate a higher-fat meal and need a pick-me-up during the two or three hours you're waiting to drink your celery juice, it's okay to have a light snack or drink some water. Just make sure to give your gut time to process them before drinking your midday celery juice. And again, wait at least 15 to 30 minutes after finishing your celery juice before consuming anything else.

Supplements and Medications

If you are on a doctor-prescribed medication, it's okay to take it either before or after your celery juice, depending on whether it's supposed to be taken on an empty stomach or with food. (Please note that if your medication is supposed to be taken with food, celery juice does not count as a food.) If you take the medication first, try to wait at least 15 to 20 minutes and ideally 30 minutes before you drink your celery juice. If you drink your celery juice first, try to wait at least 15 to 20 minutes and ideally 30 minutes before you take your medication. For any further questions or concerns, consult your physician.

If you are on supplements, please hold off on taking your supplements with your celery juice. While the supplements will do fine with the celery juice, the celery juice is better without the supplements. It's best to wait to take your supplements until at least 15 to 20 minutes and ideally 30 minutes after you've finished your celery juice.

Coffee

I'm not against drinking coffee. I'm just not for it as a health food. Coffee tends to wear down the adrenals and make the body acidic, wearing out the stomach glands as well and causing lower hydrochloric acid and eventual putrefaction of food as the years go by. This leads to ammonia gas in the gut that seeps up into the mouth and leads to dental and gum decay. It's astringent on the system, harsh on the intestinal linings and tooth enamel, and extremely dehydrating. I've heard countless times that people fear citrus such as oranges and lemons, because they're told by misinformed professionals that citrus weakens, cracks, and dissolves tooth enamel. Many of these very same people who are afraid of citrus will often drink coffee on a daily basis, and that's far more injurious to the teeth than any orange or lemon ever could be. Citrus, including oranges, lemons, limes, and grapefruit, is healthy for the teeth and gums because it's antibacterial—and bacteria is the very cause of gum disease and cavities—while also high in calcium to help strengthen teeth and the jawbone.

If you like your coffee and want to drink it because that's your vice, there are a lot worse things you can consume. It's best to drink it a minimum of 15 to 20 minutes and ideally 30 minutes *after* your celery juice. If you drink coffee before your celery juice, the juice will have to work that much harder to correct and heal what's going on in your body, and it already has enough on its plate. That said, if you need coffee first thing in the morning, before even your celery juice, I get it. At least give the coffee 15 minutes at the minimum and ideally 30 minutes or so to go through your system before drinking your celery juice. The juice will still help you in many ways; it just won't do everything it needs to do as fast as it can. Now, if you're living with a symptom or condition, do consider giving your body a break from coffee and opting for coconut water instead. Taking a vacation from coffee alone will help you feel improvements, and then the celery juice will build on that healing.

Will celery juice help break a coffee addiction? Often when we live our lives filled up with troublemakers that the body deems toxic, the reason we reach for caffeine is to trigger adrenaline to mask the effect the toxins have on us. That's all without us realizing it. Usually we have no idea how much we've been exposed to, how many poisons and pathogens have taken up residence in our livers, bloodstream, and more; we just know that we're not feeling 100 percent and that coffee keeps us going in the moment. Because celery juice helps cleanse these troublemakers, the need for adrenaline to mask them diminishes over time—which means that after a period of committing to celery juice, yes, those strong urges to knock back caffeine can dissipate for many people.

Exercise

People often wonder how they should fit celery juice into their morning workout routine. The absolute ideal scenario is to wake up, drink some lemon water, wait 15 to 30 minutes, drink your celery juice, wait another 15 to 30 minutes, eat what you like to eat before a workout (preferably a fat-free item like a fruit smoothie), give that some time to digest, and then go off to your run, hike, bike ride, tennis match, swim session, volleyball game, gym time, or whatever other exercise you like.

It's totally understandable if you don't have enough time for that. In that case, the next best option is to skip the lemon water and instead drink your celery juice first thing, wait 15 to 30 minutes, eat some breakfast (again, a fruit smoothie is ideal), give it some time to settle, and then go work out.

Both of the above options give you celery juice's empty-stomach benefits while also giving you fuel for your exercise—that is, breakfast. Remember, celery juice is not a calorie source; it's a medicinal. Athletes need calories and carbohydrates or they burn out and hit a wall. (If you believe that athletes run on protein, look into the rest of the Medical Medium series for nutritional guidance.) Celery juice alone before getting started is okay if it's only going to be light exercise. Before any vigorous exercise, though, it's a good idea to get some fuel in you, and celery juice is not fuel. The best workout food, whether before or after a workout, is a piece of fresh fruit or a fruit smoothie.

What if you're still really committed to getting in your workout first thing? Then drink your celery juice before or drink your celery juice after, or do both; it's up to you. I still advise getting some food in you before you go out so your body has fuel. If you drink celery juice when you get back, I don't advise drinking it alone. As good as celery juice is for replenishing the electrolytes, neurotransmitter chemicals, critical sodium reserves, and trace minerals you've lost through perspiration and exertion—and it can help restore these better than anything else can—you're going to hit a wall if you don't get calories, too, following intense exercise. Once you've consumed your celery juice following a workout, don't wait very long before consuming fresh fruit or another critical clean carbohydrate (CCC), explained more in Chapter 8 and *Liver Rescue*, to give yourself vital glucose. Waiting to eat your snack 5 to 10 minutes after drinking your post-workout celery juice is a good window. It's true that in this case, you won't reap every benefit of celery juice—for example, it won't be the pathogen killer that it is on its own. It will still provide that excellent electrolyte replenishment, though; you will still get some of its value.

If you're not loving the idea of missing out on some of celery juice's benefits by having it too close to food, then go back to the beginning of this section and see if there's a way to shift your morning routine to allow time for both celery juice and food spaced out before a workout. That combination has the best chance of supporting you for the long haul.

CELERY JUICE ORAL THERAPY

Once you have your fresh celery juice in hand, there are no rules about how to drink it. You can sip it. You can swish it around in your mouth for a few seconds before swallowing. Or you can send it right down. It's up to you.

When you're dealing with specific issues in and around your mouth, there are oral therapies you can use when drinking your celery juice. If you're an oil pulling enthusiast, know that celery juice for oral and dental issues is unmatched. Try switching out oil pulling for rinsing with and swallowing celery juice. How much you use these techniques depends on the severity of your condition. For a mild condition, you can try these once or more per glass. For a more severe condition, you can try one of these therapies three times or more per glass. Here they are:

- If you're exhibiting a sore throat, you can keep a sip of celery juice in your mouth for 30 seconds, letting it sit toward the back of the throat so it can kill the bacteria or virus creating the soreness. Try gargling, too, if you'd like.

- If you have swollen glands in your throat or neck, you can keep it in the back of your mouth, toward the throat, for a full minute before swallowing to help drive it into your lymphatic system over time.

- If you're dealing with tonsil stones, you can do a gentle gargle with celery juice before swallowing.

- If you have a canker sore or ulcer in your mouth, try first drying off the sore or ulcer with a paper towel or tissue and then taking a sip of your celery juice that you hold in your mouth, making sure that it covers the sensitive spot, for 30 seconds or longer before swallowing.

- If you have a toothache or tooth abscess, or if you have an injury in your mouth (for example, from biting the inside of your lip or cheek) let a sip of celery juice sit in your mouth for 30 to 60 seconds to help those sodium cluster salts enter the trouble spot and do their healing.

- If you've had a tooth pulled, you can leave a sip of celery juice in your mouth for 15 to 30 seconds—don't swish, though—and then swallow.

- If you have a cavity, slowly sip the whole glass of celery juice, giving each one a gentle swish around the mouth. (This is an exception to the guidance above about how many times to use these therapies per glass. In this case, do swish with every sip.)

- If you have receding gums or any kind of gum disease, you can gently swish a sip of celery juice around in your mouth for one minute and then swallow.

- If you have a cold sore, fever blister, or bacterial infection of any kind on the lip, you can let the celery juice touch it, using your finger to dab if needed, and then keep a sip in your mouth for 30 to 60 seconds before swallowing.

- If you get cracks in the corners of your mouth, sip your celery juice slowly and let it find its way into those painful crevices—this can help them heal much more quickly. If you have chapped or cracked lips, you can also sip your celery juice in such a way that you let some coat your lips. In either case, you can also use your finger to dab your lips or corners of your mouth with the celery juice, if that's easier.

PREGNANCY AND BREASTFEEDING

Celery juice is very safe to consume during both pregnancy and breastfeeding. During pregnancy, it helps strengthen the mother's adrenal glands, and that's critical for helping the baby, as giving birth requires large supplies of adrenaline. Strong adrenals prepare a mother to deliver her baby safely—adrenaline is what creates the "push"—and can even lead to less time in labor. Celery juice is also rich in nutrients such as vitamin K, folate, and vitamin A, all of which are important for babies' development. Its abundant antioxidants help protect babies' cells while they're developing in the womb, arming them with the ability to fight off toxins to help prevent early illness. Celery juice's sodium cluster salts also provide a developing baby's brain with neurotransmitter chemicals to support this critical phase.

During breastfeeding, a mother's consumption of celery juice is very nourishing for the baby. You don't need to worry that the detox celery juice brings about will lead to toxins in the breast milk. Quite the opposite. A woman's breast milk is usually filled with a variety of toxins to begin with, since so many people's livers are sluggish, stagnant, and overburdened from a lifetime of exposure to toxic heavy metals such as mercury and aluminum, pesticides, herbicides, fungicides, petrochemicals, cosmetics, solvents, hair dye, colognes, perfumes, and more. When these troublemakers build up in the liver, they tend to end up in the breast milk. Now, when celery juice is on the scene, its powerful components also end up in the breast milk, and they defuse, disarm, and disable the toxins—neutralizing them so that they're less destructive and even helping remove some of these toxins from the breast milk altogether. At the same time celery juice helps create clean breast milk, it provides its critical sodium cluster salts for the baby's brain development as well as viable vitamins, trace minerals, and other nutrients to keep the baby healthy.

So celery juice is very supportive for both pregnancy and breastfeeding. (And as you read in Chapter 3, "Relief from Your Symptoms and Conditions," it's even helpful *before* conception, helping address the underlying causes of infertility.) What isn't so safe is the host of different food chemicals such as citric acid and natural flavors in packaged foods, the aspartame in diet sodas, the caffeine in coffee and black tea, the antibiotics in some animal products, and harsh toxic salts that are added to so many foods, and yet these are often ingested while someone is pregnant or breastfeeding. The last thing you need to worry about is celery juice.

CELERY JUICE FOR PETS

People often feel so great when they're on celery juice that they wonder if they can give it to their pets, too. Celery juice is safe for dogs and cats, and I can even tell you that I use it personally for my dogs. Check with your vet for what amount is right for

your particular dog or cat. If you're interested in giving celery juice to another type of animal, ask your vet about whether it's appropriate.

CELERY ALLERGIES

There's a big difference between an allergy test showing a sensitivity to celery and somebody actually experiencing an immediate allergic reaction to celery. Food sensitivity testing is not always accurate. When certain foods help rid you of toxins and poisons and kill off viruses and bacteria, they tend to register falsely as allergies or sensitivities on tests.

Celery juice does indeed kill off viruses and bacteria in your system. In the process, viral and bacterial cells essentially explode, which releases whatever fuel sources were inside the pathogens, keeping them alive. That pathogenic fuel comes from a variety of foods, including eggs, dairy products, and gluten that you've eaten, along with toxic heavy metals that have entered your system. Part of what confuses allergy tests are these released viral and bacterial food particles floating through the bloodstream on the way out of the body. The pathogenic die-off that celery juice prompts will also send viral waste matter such as neurotoxins and dermatoxins into the bloodstream for eventual elimination, and this can interfere with allergy tests results, too. Food allergy testing is still in its beginning stages; it remains inconclusive. The effects of all this die-off can make you think that you're having an allergic reaction to a food or medicinal such as celery juice, when what it's really doing is clearing out unproductive bugs.

If the only reason you're avoiding celery juice is because you once had a food allergy test that suggested a sensitivity—and not because you've ever had an actual reaction to celery—you will most likely find that drinking celery juice long term changes the results of that test. Again, when someone's liver is filled with toxic chemicals and pathogens, their blood becomes toxic, and that throws off food sensitivity testing. As you drink celery juice, you will be cleaning up your liver and eliminating the very pathogens such as EBV, shingles, cytomegalovirus, herpes simplex, HHV-6, *E. coli*, strep, and staph, as well as toxins, that trigger positives on food sensitivity tests and gene mutation tests. In turn, that will allow for more accurate test results in the future that will probably no longer indicate a celery sensitivity. I've witnessed this many times over the years, where after consuming celery juice for a while, test results don't show an allergy anymore.

What if someone has an immediate allergic reaction to celery or celery juice itself? Two things could be happening. First, celery juice could be gently shocking to the system, quickly killing off bugs or even certain varieties of unproductive fungus high up in the digestive tract, in the mouth or stomach. When that happens, as we just touched on, what someone's really experiencing is a pathogenic die-off reaction rather than an allergy to the herb itself. You'll read more about detox reactions like this in Chapter 6, "Healing and Detox Answers." In these cases, you can switch over to pure cucumber juice for a while instead (see Chapter 9, "Alternatives to Celery Juice"). While cucumber juice is not a replacement for what celery juice can offer, it can gently clean the liver and gut, at least starting you off and gradually getting you to a point where you can graduate to using the awesome power of celery juice. If you want to try celery juice, try it in very small amounts and only increase if you can tolerate it. It's okay to stop periodically, take small breaks, and start over again.

Then there's the second possibility: a true celery allergy. There are those few people on the planet for whom this is the case. If your reactions to celery are severe, please continue to avoid celery and celery juice. Stick with the alternatives from Chapter 9.

Lastly, you might have heard that celery isn't great for anyone because it's a hybrid food, and this somehow makes it less natural or healthful for us to consume. If that's a concern for you, turn to Chapter 7, "Rumors, Concerns, and Myths" to read about how very natural and beneficial hybridization (not to be confused with genetic modification) can be.

INTERMITTENT FASTING

Is it okay to drink celery juice while fasting? I'm not against it. It's all about what you want to do. In the case of intermittent fasting, it's often not true fasting anyway.

Instead, you're usually limiting calories for the day or only eating during a certain part of the day. Your body only goes into a fasting mode after a full sun cycle; that is, after 24 hours of consuming no food whatsoever and only water. What's known as "intermittent fasting" could more accurately be called "intermittent eating" or "intermittent food withholding." During this, your body is not in actual fasting mode. Celery juice can be incorporated anywhere within your intermittent fasting program. (Even if you were on an actual fast, it wouldn't hurt to drink celery juice.)

Please be aware that when you're consuming celery juice, you're not consuming food. It's not providing calories. While yes,

celery has a few calories, they're not enough for your body to recognize celery juice as a calorie source. Plan accordingly—don't count on celery juice to fuel you.

THE NEXT LEVEL

This chapter has been all about how to make celery juice work for you. Before that, you discovered why celery juice even matters by exploring where it came from, what makes it the herbal medicine of our time, and how it can help people suffering from a myriad of health problems get their lives back. Now let's take it to the next level by examining how to make celery juice work *even better* for you.

CHAPTER 5

The Celery Juice Cleanse

For celery juice to work even better, you can take some simple extra steps to turn it into a true cleanse. Let's go over them:

30 DAYS OR MORE

First, you need to commit to at least a full month of drinking celery juice every day when you get up—while also following the other suggestions in this chapter for those 30 days or more. That's important. We tend to have a lot that needs to be addressed in our bodies. We've got the old, caked, rancid fats and hardened proteins on the intestinal linings; the sluggish, stagnant livers filled with pesticides, pharmaceuticals, plastics, other petroleum, stored toxic fats, pathogens such as viruses and bacteria, and more; toxic acids from the gut all the way up to the mouth; high blood toxicity and elevated blood fat; plus the state of chronic dehydration in which most people live. Then there are all of the pathogens sitting in our guts alone, not to mention in our bloodstreams, thyroids, and more. Remember, celery juice has a lot of fish to fry. (If you need a reminder of just how much, turn back to "Why 16 Ounces?" in the previous chapter.) We need to give celery juice a chance to perform its many jobs.

OPTIONAL LEMON OR LIME WATER

Before you drink your celery juice each morning during this cleanse, you have the option of drinking lemon or lime water (or plain water) first, upon waking. A good amount is 32 ounces. This gives the liver a cleansing first thing in the morning.

If you go this route, make sure you wait at least 15 to 20 minutes and ideally 30 minutes or so after finishing your water before you start sipping your celery juice so you don't dilute the juice in your system. Remember, adding water to your celery juice or combining the two in your stomach destroys the juice's healing abilities.

The misinformation out there claiming that celery juice is the same as water is incorrect. Celery juice clashes with water. These two liquids are even more vastly different than two worlds colliding. If you drink your lemon water and immediately follow it with celery juice, or vice versa, you'll cancel out the juice's benefits. Even if it's just a glass of plain water, it will still clash with celery juice in your system if they're not spaced out. Any time you're having water before celery juice, give it those 15 to 30 minutes or so to work through your system before you reach for celery juice.

16 OUNCES OF CELERY JUICE ON AN EMPTY STOMACH

If this is your very first time with celery juice, you don't need to start with 16 ounces. You could begin with 4 or 8 ounces and work your way up a little bit every day until you reach the full serving size.

And remember, you're not going to get the results you're looking for by eating celery sticks every day alone, throwing celery in your smoothie instead, or drinking a green juice that has celery as one of multiple ingredients. As always, we are talking about 16 ounces of pure, fresh, unadulterated celery juice. This is a case where simplest is best.

Be cautious about being derailed by the new misinformation that surfaces nearly every day about how to use celery juice. You'll find that people are trying to mix items into their celery juice, whether celery

pulp, protein powders, collagen, spices such as turmeric or cayenne, ice cubes, or fruit and vegetables juices. These concoctions, however inventive or seemingly logical, only end up hurting the people who most need healing. It's imperative that when you're applying celery juice to your life, whether in this cleanse or beyond, it be pure, straight celery juice on an empty stomach, not celery-apple juice or celery-kale juice or celery-spinach juice or any other combination. Keep it perfectly simple.

REMEMBER BREAKFAST

At least 15 to 20 minutes—and ideally a full 30 minutes or more—after finishing your celery juice, it's time to bring in some breakfast. Celery juice is a medicinal drink, not a calorie source, so you're going to need some fuel to get through the rest of your morning. Fresh fruit or a fruit smoothie are your best options. The Heavy Metal Detox Smoothie (find the recipe on page 152) makes an excellent breakfast. Oatmeal cooked in water (rather than milk) and served with or without fruit is a good option, too.

If you're concerned about fruit because you've subscribed to the fruit fear that spooks people away from eating one of the healthiest forms of food on the planet, please look into how fruit isn't responsible for poor health. Quite the opposite. Try not to be afraid of apples, raspberries, strawberries, blueberries, papayas, mangoes, melons, bananas, oranges, and so many other fruits. For help with this, turn to the "Fruit

Fear" chapter in *Medical Medium* and the entire fruit section of *Life-Changing Foods*.

FAT-FREE MORNING

Whatever you choose to eat over the course of the morning, make sure that it's free of radical fats. Foods that get their calories from fat (including nuts, peanut butter, seeds, oil, coconut, eggs, nut milk, soy milk, dairy milk, butter, cream, cheese, yogurt, other dairy, chicken, meat, fish, fish oil capsules, bacon, sausage, and ham) will hold back your healing if you turn to them at this point in the day.

(If you work a night shift, then take "morning" to mean those first several hours after you've woken up in the afternoon or evening. Keep your eating free of radical fats between when you start your day with celery juice and when you eat your midday meal, whatever the middle of your day is.)

As soon as you eat or drink radical fats, your liver must switch over to producing ample bile to send to your intestinal tract to help you digest and disperse them. On top of which, your liver must process fat that's entering the organ through the bloodstream and also store some of the fats so the heart doesn't get bombarded with too high an elevation of blood fat. All of this interrupts your body's natural morning cleanse state.

Even when you have a weakened liver, when you dump any fats into the stomach, your liver will overwork itself to deliver some bile to help you. Any bile that your liver releases, even if it's diminished, is still going to interfere with celery juice working for you. Also, when a liver is in this weakened state, being forced to produce bile generates liver heat, and that liver heat can diminish the power of celery juice further because it weakens celery juice's enzymes. Liver heat also forces the body to rush blood from the extremities to the digestive tract, and all that blood on the scene dilutes celery juice's sodium cluster salts as they're trying to kill pathogens residing within the blood vessels in the linings of the intestinal tract.

Further, if your liver is forced to release a large amount of bile in the morning, the bile dilutes celery juice's sodium cluster salts, digestive enzymes, and plant hormones that are still doing their job in your gut and the rest of your body. Drinking celery juice on an empty stomach with no fats, and then staying fat-free for a few hours after that, leaves room for the sodium cluster salts to eat up and dissolve pathogens, toxic acid, and mucus in the gut as well as old, rancid, hardened, caked-on fats and proteins from the digestive tract linings—problems that are behind symptoms and conditions such as SIBO, diverticulitis, celiac disease, colitis, bloating, and constipation. With fats in the morning diet, celery juice can lose its opportunity to kill off these bugs, raise hydrochloric acid to benefit digestion, and restore the liver. Once a rush of bile is on the scene, the gut's focus will become using that bile to break down fats that are being consumed in the moment. If radical fats aren't present, celery juice can go to work.

When people mix their celery juice with avocado, protein powders (even pea or rice protein), collagen, or anything similar, again, it forces the liver to produce extra morning bile, and that interferes with what the celery juice's sodium cluster salts are supposed to be doing to address past damage all along the alimentary canal. Same goes for consuming those fat and protein sources too soon after celery juice. To give your celery juice a chance to do all of its jobs, stay away from radical fats until at least lunchtime and fill up on nourishing, fortifying fruit, with leafy greens if desired. Oatmeal is another handy option. Later in the morning, some steamed potatoes, sweet potatoes, or winter squash could hit the spot, too. Remember, no nuts, seeds, nut butters, oils, avocados, or animal proteins.

AVOID PROBLEMATIC FOODS

Throughout the whole day, for all 30-plus days, try to avoid the following foods. You'll find much more information on why these don't serve your healing throughout the Medical Medium series:

- Milk, cheese, butter, whey protein powder, yogurt, and all other dairy products

- Eggs

- Gluten

- Corn

- Soy

- Pork products

- Nutritional yeast

- Canola oil

- Natural flavors

- Vinegar

- Fermented foods

RECAP

That's it. That's the whole cleanse. For at least 30 days:

- Optional: Drink 32 ounces of lemon or lime water upon waking, then wait 15 to 30 minutes

- Drink your celery juice (working up to 16 ounces) on an empty stomach every morning, and then wait 15 to 30 minutes before you . . .

- Enjoy a fat-free breakfast (ideally fruit, a fruit smoothie such as the Heavy Metal Detox Smoothie [see page 152], or oatmeal cooked in water)

- Keep avoiding radical fats (including milk, cheese, butter, eggs, oil, peanut butter, and more) until at least lunchtime

- Stay hydrated for the whole day

- Avoid the problematic foods all day for all 30 days

You're likely to find that you feel so great, you want to keep going past 30 days. People suffering with chronic health issues often benefit from longer than a month, because they have more to heal and repair. We'll go over the timing of healing more in the next chapter, "Healing and Detox Answers."

If you want even more advanced and significant healing, turn to Chapter 8, "More Healing Guidance," where you'll find some of the key recommendations from the Medical Medium series distilled. In my books *Thyroid Healing* and *Liver Rescue*, you'll also find more comprehensive cleanses that incorporate celery juice. As powerful as celery juice is, and even as powerful as this Celery Juice Cleanse is, nothing compares to combining the force of celery juice with other healing protocols that come from the same source.

What if you launch into this cleanse and then find one day that you can't get celery or celery juice? It happens—you can't control if there was a storm hundreds of miles away that temporarily interrupted your local grocer's supply of celery or if the juice counters in the area are sold out. In cases like these, turn to Chapter 9, "Alternatives to Celery Juice," to get yourself through the interruption.

That chapter will also help you out if you're one of the few people who can't do celery at all. For your cleanse, select one of the alternatives listed there and apply it to your life as though it were celery juice while also following the other guidance in this chapter.

If you can do celery juice, though, do. Plan ahead by ordering a weekly case of celery from your local grocer if needed. Scope out the stores in your area that stock it so you know where to turn if your regular shop is out of it. If you'll be traveling, research juice spots ahead of time or even consider bringing your juicer along for the ride. Your commitment will pay off.

Finally, as you go through your cleanse, you may find that certain symptoms arise temporarily as your body detoxes. Don't lose heart. That's natural, and we'll cover what to expect and what it means in the next chapter.

While the Celery Juice Cleanse may seem basic and easy, don't let the simplicity fool you. This isn't an ants-on-a-log snack from third grade. This is an herbal medicine, and you're consuming a large quantity of the extraction every day. Be not only open to the power it holds; be mindful of what you possess when you're holding this herbal tonic in your hands. Respect it and honor it for what it is rather than being swayed by what you thought it was. Don't be deceived by the disregard for celery that has been instilled in us through the years.

Keep in mind what it has done for so many already. Keep in mind their conditions and symptoms and illnesses, their heartfelt stories of struggle and pain and disease reversal, and their awe at the glory of recovery. Keep these individuals in your heart, too. You may soon be looking for that same validation of your healing story—of what you went through before, and what it took to get here. You, too, may be looking for people to receive and respect your testimonial so that this information can be passed along to help others heal.

"Be mindful of what you possess
when you're holding this herbal tonic in your hands.
Respect it and honor it for what it is."

— Anthony William, Medical Medium

CHAPTER 6

Healing and Detox Answers

How long will it take to feel better from celery juice? That depends. How many ounces are you on? Are you drinking it on an empty stomach? Have you stuck with it every day? What else are you doing besides celery juice—are you incorporating other Medical Medium healing advice? All these intricacies matter when it comes to the timing of feeling better.

Some people start to see benefits within three days. Some people see benefits within a week or two. I've even seen many people benefit in one day. The first benefits could be a feeling of calm or peacefulness, less anxiousness, or a boost in energy. That's because celery juice's electrolytes have an illuminating effect on mood. Many people quickly experience smoother digestion and better elimination from celery juice's digestive enzymes. If you're still struggling after a couple of weeks, that's normal, too. Everyone has different health situations for celery juice to address, so the amount of time it takes to do that varies.

People sometimes ask how long they're supposed to keep celery juice in their lives. The answer is that we should never put a timeline on drinking celery juice. How long into your life do you plan on wearing socks? The dream home you hope to purchase—how long do you plan to live there? How long do you want to be with your soul mate? How far into the future do you plan on keeping up with your favorite pastimes? Going to the beach, sailing, tennis, karaoke—do you plan on giving these up someday? Some parts of our lives—the ones that help us emotionally, physically, spiritually, and mentally—we never want to let go. Celery juice should be one of them. It's not a vitamin that you take for a month and then never again. It's a longstanding passion to cherish your whole life.

That's not to say that you're chained to a juicer every day for the rest of your life. Interruptions to taking care of yourself and doing the right thing always come. The juicer could break down. A juice bar around the corner could close. Your place of work could move farther away from the grocery store that stocks the best celery. You could get intensely busy on a project. You could go on a trip where celery or celery juice is impossible to find. It's exactly what happens to us with our other important avocations and relationships, where sometimes we're separated for a time. It's okay, as long as we keep it in mind that we'll get back to it someday, just like we do our other loves in life.

Now, if you're someone for whom that kind of thinking doesn't work because you like clear boundaries and guidelines, or you're only willing to give celery juice a trial run, then please give celery juice on an empty stomach a try every day for a full month. If that hasn't alleviated your symptoms all the way, look into the rest of the Medical Medium series for other tools to use along with the celery juice. Keep going until you feel better.

Is it safe to keep drinking celery juice long term? Well, let's think about what "safe" means: free from harm. And let's think about what's more likely to cause harm: drinking a medicinal beverage that provides daily defense against pathogens and poisons in our everyday world, or not getting that protection? Celery juice's very job is to keep you safe—more than safe— long term. The more you use it, the more it can help you.

KEY HEALING FACTORS

If you feel like you're not seeing any benefits from celery juice, we need to dissect that a little bit. How sick were you when you started? Have you been on medications, struggling with a chronic illness, for a long time? Are you still consuming problematic foods from Chapter 8, "More Healing Guidance," that are feeding, not helping, your illness? Some people who have really struggled with their health need to work up to 16 ounces of celery juice twice a day, or 32 ounces in the morning.

If you're going to try 32 ounces or more in the morning, you don't need to gulp it all down in 5 or even 10 minutes. Everyone consumes beverages at a different pace. Some like to sip gently and mindfully. Some are working while they're sipping, and they get distracted. Some are taking it on the go. Within reason, take the time you need to drink your larger serving of celery juice. Ideally, get it all down within an hour. If you stretch past that, sporadically taking sips throughout the whole morning and eating in between, it will interrupt the juice's healing benefits. If you sporadically take sips throughout the whole morning and don't eat anything, you could end up feeling faint or cranky because you didn't get any meaningful calories over those several hours.

The effects of celery juice can feel different every day. Sometimes people develop detox symptoms—that is, healing reactions—when they start on celery juice.

Sometimes they witness amazing healing benefits. There may be times when you're feeling great and times when you're still suffering or struggling. You can't mistake the down times for celery juice letting you down. Throughout it all, you'll still be moving forward.

If one day you don't feel much of a difference in any direction, that doesn't mean it's not doing anything. A day when it doesn't seem to be "working" could be a day when celery juice is busy getting junk out of your liver, replenishing cells throughout your body, rebuilding your immune system, helping your kidneys, correcting your endocrine system, and repairing your digestive tract—and then you may feel the healing effects of that detox later in the week, month, or even year. With commitment over time, more and more good days will come as celery juice has less and less to fix.

Your liver's state of health when you start drinking celery juice has a big effect on how long it takes to see improvements. So does your diet. It's common for people to be on a high-fat diet without realizing it—thinking it's only high in protein and not knowing that the constant high levels of fat are undermining their health. As I covered in *Liver Rescue*, high-protein diets are high-fat diets, too, even if we're talking about healthy fats and proteins such as avocados, seeds, nut butters, olives, olive oil, and lean, grass-fed, free-range meats. Too much of any type of fat, bad or good, leads to a bloodstream thick with fat, meaning that toxins can't be cleansed from the body as easily, nor can nutrients be delivered as effectively. This weighs against what celery juice can do for you and how fast it can help. It *will* still be helping, although much of that assistance will be directed at keeping up with everything the body is up against in the moment. Ideally, you want to give your body a break from the onslaught of high-fat foods and other troublemakers so that celery juice can address and repair the older issues that are holding you back.

Everyone has different levels of toxins, poisons, and pathogens in the body. Some people have multiple viruses inside the liver such as Epstein-Barr, HHV-6, and herpes simplex. Some people have colonies of bacteria such as strep and *E. coli* inside the liver and intestinal tract. Some people have been battling chlamydia through the years. Some people have a higher level of staph. Some people are dealing with undiagnosed levels of *H. pylori* in the small intestinal tract's duodenum. Some people are high in toxic heavy metals such as mercury, copper, aluminum, nickel, cadmium, lead, or barium. Some people have gotten a lot of radiation exposure from frequent airplane travel, lots of dental work, X-rays, or CT scans. Some people's livers have old storage bins of DDT passed on from earlier generations. Some people's digestive systems are loaded with insecticides and other pesticides from treatments around their home or local park. Some people even have much or all of this going on at once.

(If you're confused about what causes your symptoms or illness, immerse yourself in the Medical Medium series so you can learn about what's truly ailing you. For the millions who are suffering with autoimmune disease, for example, a viral load is responsible, so it's critical to know how to address this underlying cause directly. Without this knowledge, it's easy to accidentally feed any viruses or bacteria present in your body.)

Celery juice is like a cleaning service, and asking how long it will take is like asking that service for an estimate before anyone has seen how big a mess lies behind the door. Is the cleaning service entering a tidy office, where the job is to empty a few trash cans, vacuum lightly, and wipe the counter of the kitchenette? Or is the cleaning service walking into the aftermath of a children's birthday party, with piles of crumpled gift wrap, something sticky in the carpet, and cake smeared on the walls? Your system's particular brew of toxins and pathogens, and the particular level of suffering that brew has created, affect how long it takes to feel better. There's also an emotional component that celery juice addresses—add all of the difficult emotions that have built up along with the sickness, hardships, or challenges you've been through, and celery juice could have a lot of work in front of it. We've got to give it a chance.

I've seen people who were on celery juice for a year, at which point they miraculously started to heal on many different levels. I've also seen people who didn't realize how much healing they were doing on celery juice until they went off it. Many of us are too busy to be fully mindful and aware, and it can take stopping celery juice to wake up to how much it was helping. Some people won't even realize celery juice was a remedy. They'll stop drinking it for one reason or another, start exhibiting symptoms, and visit their practitioner asking for advice—not making the connection that going back on celery juice would put them back on track for healing.

In many cases, for example with acid reflux, a short while on celery juice can take care of the problem, and you can move on. Here's why you'd still want to consider sticking with celery juice even after it solved your current health problem: you don't want something else to go wrong down the road. The constant exposure in our lives is real. We have pollutants in our water; we encounter toxic heavy metals from aluminum foil, aluminum cans, and eating out at restaurants where all day, utensils scrape the bottoms of copper and steel pans; viruses and bacteria come at us from countless directions; and so many other varying degrees of pathogens and pollutants enter our lives on a regular basis without our knowledge or permission. If you think you'll never pick up a bacterial strain or a virus or breathe in poor quality air for the rest of your days, I'm sorry to say that's mistaken. (For a primer on what we encounter from day to day, check out the "Liver Troublemakers" chapter in *Liver Rescue*.) All of these exposures, especially when combined, can lead to health problems before too long. If you keep drinking celery juice even after your acid reflux or other problem has healed, you could spare yourself from experiencing worse later.

DON'T BLAME THE SCAPEGOAT

It's easy for celery juice to become a scapegoat. Try not to let it be one for you. That is, should a doctor or any other practitioner in the healing arts try to pin your problems on the fact that you drink celery juice, be cautious.

Healing can take a bit of time. While some symptoms can improve quickly once you start drinking celery juice, other symptoms take more time to pass because they're caused by toxins such as the toxic heavy metals mercury and aluminum, as well as pathogens such as EBV and shingles that are a little deeper-seated in the liver, thyroid, and other areas of the body—and therefore require more cleanup. Not to mention that sometimes while people are drinking celery juice, they're still eating unproductive foods or engaging in other practices that undermine celery juice's effectiveness. So, if you're a short ways into your Celery Juice Cleanse, or you're drinking it and then following it up with bacon and eggs, and you visit a doctor while still experiencing any chronic symptoms, you could hear, "The reason you're not feeling well is because you're drinking celery juice."

It's a well-meaning conclusion. Chronic symptoms and illness are a mystery to medical research and science, so medical communities are always looking for what could be behind them in order to help patients. Many practitioners are open-minded about unconventional remedies that they can see are making their patients better. Many others may see celery juice as a source of ridiculousness or confusion. It's natural to be skeptical of celery juice. Only in recent years has it received public attention, so it seems new, disconcerting, and maybe even a little spooky. Still, it's not an answer to what's behind chronic health issues. It's an answer to *how to heal* chronic health issues. Don't let celery juice become a scapegoat for the unproductive sources that do keep people sick. Don't let lack of understanding about celery juice sabotage you from accessing the very remedy that can help you recover and even save your life.

HEALING REACTIONS

Let's take a look at some of the most common healing reactions that can come with drinking celery juice so that you can understand what's going on beneath the surface. You won't necessarily experience any of these signs of detox, and that's fine, too. It means you probably have less internal cleanup work. You'll still be detoxing, even if you don't feel it.

It can sometimes be tough to discern healing reactions from symptoms caused by other sources. If, for example, everything is going along fine for months of drinking celery juice and then one day you get incredibly nauseated out of the blue, is that a healing reaction or a sudden stomach bug? Answer: a sudden stomach bug. You can use the timing of symptoms as a clue. Healing reactions to celery juice are more likely to happen when you first start drinking it, and they range from mild to undetectable.

Healing reactions are also temporary. If after one month of drinking 16 ounces of celery juice on an empty stomach every day, your issue hasn't shown any movement at all, that's an indication that it's a symptom of an underlying problem, not a healing reaction to celery juice. Consider studying Chapter 3 and digging into the rest of the Medical Medium series to learn more about the cause of your chronic issue so you can bring in more healing tools, some of which you'll find in Chapter 8, "More Healing Guidance." Celery juice alone can't tackle every problem—sometimes it needs backup.

It's okay if celery juice brings on such rapid cleansing that you're not ready to drink 16 ounces yet. It's okay to drink 4 or 6 or 8 ounces until you can work your way up. It's okay to stop and start all over again, too. It's okay to take small breaks. It's more about the long-term picture.

Remember: through it all, whether you're feeling down or up, exhausted or energetic, doubtful or hopeful, celery juice is always working for you. Hang in there with it, and it will more than hang in there with you—it will pull you through.

Now let's get into the possible healing reactions that can occur when you start celery juice. Understanding how your body is benefitting will help you stay the course.

Acid Reflux

When people develop temporary acid reflux, it's because celery juice is killing bacteria and flushing out toxins. The intestinal tract is sometimes filled with dangerous funguses, pathogens, and rancid fats baked and caked onto its linings, with proteins rotting inside of it. There's also that tiny ledge just before the duodenum that can get covered with sludge. When you're young, the sludge is practically nonexistent. As you get older, the weight of built-up residue and debris starts to press downward on the ledge, making a slight divot in some people who are overeating diets with larger amounts of animal products, even including seemingly "lighter" options such as eggs, fish, and dairy. Enough debris weighing on this divot makes a tiny pouch at the bottom of the stomach that ends up holding old, decayed matter.

As you drink celery juice, it travels down the alimentary canal, and its enzymes start hitting the mucus that goes along with the presence of all these troublemakers. Its sodium cluster salts start hitting old, rancid fats, toxins, bacteria, viruses, and funguses—breaking them down and killing them off. Celery juice also starts clearing the tiny ledge at the entrance to the duodenum and the tiny accompanying pouch of old sludge. In turn, a mini explosion occurs. Acid reflux can be the result of that die-off explosion from celery juice's massive cleanup job. (Alternatively for some, a quick bout of diarrhea can result.) Once you get past this, you're likely to start seeing huge healing benefits.

Bloating

Most often, celery juice is alleviating bloat, not causing it. If someone's liver is toxic, stagnant, and sluggish enough, though, with enough unproductive bacteria in the intestinal tract, too, then they could experience some bloating as celery juice kills off bacteria and revitalizes the liver. This would most likely be the result of drinking a larger quantity of celery juice, which tends to do deeper cleaning. Before long, someone who experiences this will usually start to find that celery juice helps reduce bloating instead.

Body Odor

A common healing reaction to celery juice is increased body odor. This odor can be produced anywhere on the skin, not only under the armpits. It happens in part because of the sluggish, stagnant livers everyone is dealing with to some degree; as the liver receives celery juice's components, the organ can release an increased amount of toxins that surface to the skin. Celery juice also disperses ammonia from rotting proteins and undigested fats inside the small intestinal tract and colon. And as celery juice is traveling through the digestive tract and lymphatic system, it can purge and expel a multitude of poisons and toxins. At the same time, celery juice disperses pockets of stored adrenaline from stressful situations that our organs have taken on, and this old adrenaline will start surfacing to the skin, too. Any or all of this can result in some variety of increased body odor. As someone gets healthier by using celery juice, eventually less body odor will occur. Celery juice can even take someone to the opposite end of the spectrum, where they experience lessened or even no body odor.

Coldness or Chills

Celery juice has a positive cooling effect on the body. When you drink it, you deliver a near-instant infusion of nutrients and phytochemical compounds to your cells and organs. Your body receiving what it needs gives it a moment of relief. This calming effect has a cooling effect—because your body is not having to overwork or struggle so much. You can experience a little chill when this happens, and it's a sign of healing as celery juice feeds every cell in your body. If you have the chance, it's a moment to grab a blanket and curl up on the couch for a minute or so to warm yourself up while celery juice is doing its healing.

Another reason you might feel a little cold when drinking celery juice is if it causes an instant detox reaction when cleaning up poisons and toxins throughout the intestinal tract. As the troublemakers are neutralized and enter the bloodstream for elimination, it can cause a slight chill.

Finally, most people's livers are running extremely hot from being imbalanced and sluggish. Celery juice cools the liver instantly, and that can cause a body temperature fluctuation.

Constipation

Celery juice does not cause constipation. If you're backed up, this is one of those times to look for another answer about what's causing it. Were you already constipated when you started drinking celery juice? Are you eating the unproductive foods from Chapter 8? Are you going through an emotional trial that has your gut tied up in knots? Over time, celery juice can help alleviate your constipation by reducing the chronic or acute inflammation that could be occurring inside your intestinal tract. Intestinal inflammation tends to cause the slowdown of peristaltic action, resulting in bouts of constipation. Celery juice helps right this.

Dry Skin

If you're using celery juice and you notice that your skin is dry, ask yourself a few questions: Has it ever been dry before? What is the weather like—is it cold, and have you been exposed to a lot of dry indoor heat? Are you bathing in chlorinated water? Has anything changed in your diet that could be leading to dry skin? Keep in mind that it can take time for your diet to show its effects on your skin, so don't just think back to the last couple of days. Has anything changed in your diet within the last couple of months? If nothing else accounts for your dry skin—if this is the first time you've ever experienced it, your indoor or outdoor environment doesn't account for it and neither does anything you've been using on it or exposed to topically, and your diet has remained steady for months—then dry skin can be a sign of celery juice cleansing your liver. A liver filled with petrochemicals, solvents, gasoline, perfume, cologne, pesticides,

herbicides, fungicides, toxic heavy metals, pharmaceuticals from the past, and under-the-radar viruses and other pathogens will start to detox when you drink celery juice. Many toxins will head toward the skin to be delivered out of the body, and dry skin can result temporarily, until your liver improves. With long-term use of celery juice, you can end up with better skin than ever before.

Headaches and Migraines

This is yet another case where the first step is to ask yourself if you've ever experienced this symptom before. Is this a regular occurrence, where you get headaches on and off? If so, it is possible that celery juice *triggered* the pain, although it didn't cause it. Your frequent migraines are most likely from toxic heavy metals, a low-grade viral or bacterial infection, or a liver overrun with toxins. When you encounter a healing force such as celery juice, it can easily trigger symptoms that you deal with on a regular basis because it gets troublemakers moving on their way out of your body. For example, as celery juice kills off bugs in your body, if you're already sensitive to migraines, that could give you another migraine. You will be going in the right direction, though, toward ridding yourself of your symptoms by helping to heal the stagnant liver, toxic heavy metal load, or viral or bacterial infection that underlies what's ailing you.

If you've never had a headache or migraine in your life and you get your first one after starting celery juice, it's still not the celery juice that's causing it—you just happened to drink celery juice that day, and since it's new to you, it's getting the blame. Think about what food products could have caused your headache. MSG disguised as "natural flavors" in an herbal tea bag is a possible culprit. So is a cup of coffee spiked with a little too much caffeine. Dehydration is a big factor, too. There are many elements that can contribute to the development of headaches or migraines. Celery juice isn't one of them. Try celery juice again on a day when you avoid dehydration, food additives, and foods you don't usually eat.

Mood Shifts

Irritability, frustration, agitation: it can feel a little disconcerting to experience these emotions as celery juice is making your skin glow, giving you more energy, and freeing you from aches and pains. Not to worry. If you're feeling a little down, moody, or depressed after drinking celery juice, even alongside all its wonderful benefits, it's a normal, temporary healing reaction. You could be experiencing the detox effect of killing off viruses and bacteria and cleansing poisons. You could also be detoxing emotions—that often goes hand in hand with detoxing troublemakers. As you continue to heal, your mood will start to lift.

When someone uses celery juice as a meal replacement, it can also cause moodiness. For one, going hours without eating will cause blood sugar to drop. For another, a morning of celery juice alone will lead to faster and more erratic detoxing—which isn't recommended—and that accelerated

cleanse state can lead to extra grumpiness. Remember: after you've had your morning celery juice, follow it up at least 15 to 20 minutes and ideally 30 minutes later with a healing calorie source such as fruit. (And remember, too: don't fear fruit!)

Mouth and Tongue Sensations

People can experience varied sensations on the tongue or elsewhere in the mouth when drinking celery juice. These can include a funny feeling, tingling, or even slight numbness or burning, either generally or in a specific spot like the gums or the tip of the tongue. This indicates a higher level of bacteria or toxins in the mouth, and/or an elevated amount of ammonia in the mouth that's coming from foods putrefying in the intestinal tract, outgassing, and seeping up through the esophagus. When you drink celery juice, its sodium cluster salts collide with these rogue visitors, and it's that reaction that leads to tingling or irritation in the mouth or even the throat, if bacteria are hanging out back there.

If you experience a metallic taste or other funny flavor from celery juice and funny tastes have never happened to you before, this is a detox reaction occurring. It means that celery juice has entered your liver and is starting to flush out a variety of troublemakers—anything from pesticides to herbicides to fungicides to petrochemicals to solvents, as well as toxic heavy metals themselves. Celery juice also has the ability to flush heavy metals' oxidative material from throughout the body's organs and tissues. Some people have heavy metals in their guts, in which case, celery juice will help bind onto and expel them from the system. Any and all of these can have an effect on taste. Whether that's a metallic taste or another unusual flavor varies depending on someone's particular toxic brew.

Nausea and Vomiting

Some slight nausea after drinking celery juice can be an indication of a little healing pathogenic die-off and detox.

If you're vomiting after drinking it, that's most likely an indication that you were exposed to something else that's unrelated. Millions of people are drinking celery juice globally. A small percentage of them could happen to get food poisoning, catch a stomach flu, or be exposed to a toxic substance—which means that a small percentage of people are going to have a throw-up day that coincides with drinking celery juice. Because celery juice seems like an oddball, it's apt to take the blame.

If you are one of the rare few for whom everything was in perfect working order—no sensitive stomach, no bugs, no chemical exposure—until you drank your celery juice, and then you immediately threw up, then it could have been a gag reflex due to a strong, bitter batch of celery. This is especially true if it was a very leafy batch of celery picked up at a local farm or farmers' market or grown at home, with leaves puffed up like a peacock. If you're juicing more leaves than stalks (which, I mentioned in Chapter 4, I don't recommend), you can

end up with a very astringent batch of juice, where the alkaloids trigger the gag reflex if you're sensitive.

Even more rarely, you could have a whole bunch of acid and bacteria or other microorganisms in the duodenum that shouldn't be there (such as undiagnosed *H. pylori*), with celery juice causing an instant die-off. I call this *radical die-off*: a large amount of bacteria or other bugs basically explode at one time, and this can trip the vagus nerve, which leads to vomiting. It is extremely infrequent that someone has enough bacteria and is sensitive enough at the same time to cause this reaction.

Rashes, Itching, and Breakouts

If this is truly an isolated response—where you're not experiencing a skin problem due to a new coffee you tried, a new fermented food you had for the first time, pesticides from your neighbor's yard that blew over to yours, brand-new clothes that you tried on without washing, or similar factors—and it can only be traced to celery juice, first make sure you're not getting your celery juice from a juice counter that washes its produce with a drop of chlorine or bleach. This is a practice that certain natural food stores and juice shops do use that will not mean good things for your health, so be sure to ask how your celery juice is prepared and find a new spot if they use this technique. Also, if the juice bar you're visiting uses conventional celery rather than organic, it's almost better to go get some conventional celery, if that's what you can access or afford, and make the juice yourself, because then you can make sure you're washing it well to avoid any pesticide exposure.

If you've ruled out all of the above and you weren't exposed to anything new and irritating that could be causing your rash, itching, or breakout, then it means you have a large variety of troublemakers that have built up in your liver and celery juice is now cleansing them as part of its job. These could include viral waste matter such as byproduct, neurotoxins, and dermatoxins, the last of which especially affect the skin as they rise up through it. Celery juice's sodium cluster salts also find their way up through the dermis, where they help neutralize and detox these poisons from the skin.

Thirst

If you experience pronounced thirst after drinking celery juice, this is because celery juice is cleansing and detoxing poisons and flushing them out of your bloodstream. Choose the liquids that you use to quench this thirst wisely. Consider the options from the final chapter, such as lemon water and ginger water, to drink later on, once you've had your celery juice and given your body a chance to process it.

Weight Loss

People are not always looking to lose weight. If your weight is where you want it to be, or if you are underweight, you don't need to worry that celery juice will make you lose body mass. The reason that celery juice helps people who are overweight reduce the pounds on the scale is that it makes their livers healthier. A healthy liver leads to balance; it helps take you where you need to be, in whatever direction that is. If you're underweight with an unhealthy liver, celery juice won't make you lose weight.

The only way celery juice can make you lose weight when that's unwelcome is if you're using celery juice as a calorie source and meal replacement. If you are, you're replacing the hundreds of calories that you would get from a meal with the handful of calories that you get from celery juice. This prolonged calorie reduction can cause someone who easily loses weight to lose more weight. Remember, celery juice is a medicine. It's not a food. Don't accidentally deprive yourself of the calories you need by using celery juice as a stand-in for a snack or meal.

YOUR HEALING STORY

One argument that's been made to undermine celery juice is that the vast number of healing stories from people who have applied it to their lives only constitutes anecdotal evidence about its effectiveness. What about the people who are getting better from celery juice right now? What the sources who dismiss celery juice as anecdotal don't realize is that in doing so, they are invalidating people's stories. They are dismissing thousands upon thousands of people's testimonials of recovery. This disrespects those who have been chronically ill. It communicates that their perception of having been sick, tried everything to get better, and then finally found a true remedy when they brought in celery juice is somehow not to be trusted.

Don't let this disrespect shake your trust in your own healing process. Some people start drinking celery juice, change nothing else, and feel better. For other people, celery juice brings them to a certain point, and then they need more healing information from this same source to keep feeling better. Whichever it ends up being for you, know that your symptoms were real, they weren't in your head, they weren't your fault, you didn't attract them by thinking bad thoughts, and you didn't somehow deserve them as punishment. As you learned in Chapter 3, "Relief from Your Symptoms and Conditions," your health issues had actual physiological causes from this tough world that we inhabit.

Know, too, that as you start to feel improvements from celery juice, that's just as real. Don't let echoes of "anecdotal" make you doubt your recovery. You are the greatest expert on your health, and your healing story counts. It counts for more than you know. So stay strong. Someone out there right now is waiting to hear your story so they can discover this life-changing medicine.

CHAPTER 7

Rumors, Concerns, and Myths

People who have struggled with their health tend to hold pure hearts full of good intentions. They know what it's like to suffer. They've sometimes felt that medical science or the medical industry has let them down as they've searched and searched for remedies. Celery juice is the perfect match for their honesty and purity of heart. It has nothing to do with the green juice trend— it's elevated above it. Celery juice is a gift from the heavens, from God. Or if you prefer to think of it another way, it's a gift from the Universe. It's a gift from the Earthly Mother.

Those who haven't known the serious suffering of being held back in life can find it easy to make fun of celery juice. If someone has only dealt with minor, passing symptoms, it's all too simple to say that this is just another silly trend. Don't let the jokes get to you. Making fun of celery juice is, in a sense, making fun of people who've struggled with their health. It's knocking this remedy out of the hands of those who need it. As we established at the end of the previous chapter, it's disrespectful to the growing number of people who have already recovered with celery juice. It's telling them they weren't as sick as they thought to begin with and that they didn't find a safe and natural solution that brought their life back. It's telling them they're wrong.

It's also questioning their heart, their intelligence, their discernment of truth, and their intentions. That's very painful. It's like bullying them out of their own reality. As if their hard work and healing accomplishments don't matter to the world. It's like they never happened.

Over the decades, chronic illness sufferers have fought to be taken seriously. With the birth of the Internet age, they've been respected a little more because they've gotten a chance to connect and find strength in numbers. They're still not respected enough. The staggering number of people falling ill today with intermittent or chronic symptoms that cause lower quality of life is by far the highest rate in history. Those who don't recognize that or aren't shaken by it can't imagine what it's like to struggle with neurological fatigue, chronic pain, or multiple conditions at once. They don't know what it is to wait for years for an answer, finally find some relief, and then have it doubted by naysayers who are skeptical because the origin is a man who, since age four, has been hearing advanced medical healing information from a voice above.

In addition to jokes, fear tactics are a predictable side effect of the celery juice movement. Usually, trends and fads are backed by bankroll. Not only that—people then make money off them. Trends don't need to work; we just need to think they do. Because celery juice is not a trend—it has staying power—it stands apart. It wasn't invented by an industry as a moneymaker. Running celery through a juicer doesn't turn juice bars into cash cows; those are hard businesses to run, and you can't scale fresh celery juice. The reason celery juice has taken on a life of its own is not because of greed. It's because it offers something health trends don't: results. Word spread about celery juice because the Medical Medium community put out the message far and wide when they found it actually worked.

Due to its phenomenal effectiveness, it's going to come under attack here and there. Fear will be produced, both mischievously and innocently, to try to stop people from getting what they need from celery juice. In part that's due to disillusionment. People have heard about or fallen prey to so many health claims that they no longer know what to trust. Skepticism abounds. In part the distrust surrounding celery juice comes from its purity. It's simple and it's real and it works, with only good intentions behind it, and that threatens to expose other popular health "remedies" as being not so pure, effective, or aboveboard. You won't find bone broth or collagen or kombucha tea under attack, because there are vested interests that protect them. There's money to be made there. Celery juice, on the other hand, is its own free-spirited healing modality that threatens to topple empires. In the end, no one is allowed to control it, box it up, and keep it from you.

There will be *attempts* to control celery juice. There will be efforts to capitalize off the celery juice movement. Many will want to put their own twist on celery juice by mixing in additives or turning it into a pill so they can try to steer the ship and profit from it. You're about to read about why these are ineffective approaches. Ultimately, all these tactics do is guide people back to the profound truth that pure celery juice is what works. It's imperative that we preserve the healing information about celery juice that resides in this book. Someday those same people who disregard it or distort it in the present could be turning to it to answer their prayers.

Now let's dispel the myths, fears, concerns, and rumors that may be holding you back from experiencing celery juice's blessings.

ADD-INS

The temptation is always there to complicate celery juice by mixing it with seemingly healthy add-ins. Anything that takes away from the simplicity of celery juice is misguided. Any efforts to make it more "advanced" or more "more" will only disturb what celery juice has to offer. Still, even if it becomes well known that celery juice is best by itself—that extracting celery's complex nutritional offerings as juice has already transformed it into health gold—it will be impossible to stop people from exploring their inner alchemists and attempting to improve on celery juice with extra ingredients. "What can we add in and how can we add it in?" they'll ask themselves, because it's so difficult to register that this tonic in its simplest form is at its most healing. Inevitably, this will remain an ongoing problem for years to come, and the add-in campaigns will continue. Here are two examples of what's already out there, so you know to steer clear.

Apple Cider Vinegar (ACV)

Because of the popularity of apple cider vinegar—popularity that exists *not* because it has a miraculous healing record of helping people turn around chronic illness—people have started adding it to their celery juice. This has happened without anyone stopping to consider the truth that more people don't feel better after consuming apple cider vinegar than do feel better. If you're a believer in vinegar, then yes, ACV is the healthiest vinegar to use—at other times. Keep it away from your celery juice. It's one of the swiftest ways to render your celery juice completely useless; you won't obtain a single benefit from celery juice if ACV is mixed into it. Celery juice's sodium cluster salts, digestive enzymes, and plant hormones will be instantly destroyed. Its vitamin C will be instantly rendered unusable. Celery juice's structure on the whole will be instantly spoiled. Because of money-driven interests and agendas, though, adding ACV to celery juice will keep being perpetuated as a great source of health. Don't let the arguments sway you. Instead, remind yourself that when ACV hits celery juice, it oxidizes the celery juice immediately, making it go bad. You know what it's like to open a carton of milk and go, "Oh, that went bad"? It's the same here. Preserve your celery juice's integrity and keep the ACV away from it.

Collagen

Collagen is one of the most disastrous items you can mix with celery juice. There's a huge confusion about collagen in general. Collagen is a critical aspect of the human body: It's partially responsible for keeping our skin intact. It's an important protein for connective tissue throughout the body. Without healthy collagen, we can show signs of aging quickly and we can weaken internally. This has nothing to do with *consuming* collagen. Rather, we need to *build* healthy collagen.

One of the greatest mistakes in the medical industry today is the trend encouraging people to consume supplemental collagen, thinking that it will enter our digestive tract and miraculously find its way to our skin and connective tissue and fill in for human collagen. This is yet one more theory that falls under the old belief system from hundreds and hundreds of years ago that stated that if you had an ailing kidney, you should eat an animal kidney; if you had an ailing liver, you should eat liver; if you had an ailing eyeball, you should eat a sheep's eyeball. Where did that get us? Not far! We're still living in the Dark Ages if we think that eating supplemental collagen is going to fill in for our own.

The reason trend-makers make this mistake is that the medical industry doesn't have a handle on why our collagen weakens or diminishes in the first place. The truth is that the collagen we rely on in our connective tissue and skin is created by nutrients that come from plant foods: leafy greens, fruits, and even tubers, rhizomes, and root vegetables. If we have a high toxic load, it becomes destructive to this process. The weakening of collagen throughout your body is determined by how much pathogenic material is floating around in your bloodstream and how toxic your liver is with troublemakers such as pesticides, herbicides, and fungicides.

Pesticides, herbicides, and fungicides have a direct reaction with collagen, injuring it and shrinking it. Viruses in the herpetic family (such as herpes simplex 1 and 2, EBV, shingles, cytomegalovirus, HHV-6, HHV-7, and the undiscovered HHV-10 through HHV-16) tend to release a tremendous amount of neurotoxins in the liver and other organs and glands. Some of them produce dermatoxins, too. That waste matter saturates connective tissue, which saturates collagen. The viral waste slows down the development of new collagen cells while weakening and breaking down existing healthy collagen. This can even go so far as to cause connective tissue conditions. If someone is high in toxic heavy metals, it can amplify these effects and injure collagen even more.

None of this is known by medical research and science or by the collagen suppliers of the supplement world. They don't realize that swooping in with supplemental collagen doesn't solve the above, and actually makes it worse. They don't realize that any supplemental collagen we consume turns to waste in the intestinal tract because it's not meant to be there—and it's not harmless waste. When someone consumes supplemental collagen, it actually becomes fuel—not for our body, not for our cells. It becomes fuel for the cells of viruses and bacteria. Supplemental collagen diminishes productive bacteria and feeds unproductive bacteria. Viruses such as EBV feed off supplemental animal collagen. So do other microbes such as fungus, yeast, and mold. It helps them all proliferate and expand their colonies. Be very wary of mixing collagen with celery juice.

While virus cells feeding on supplemental collagen do not release neurotoxins the way virus cells feeding on toxic heavy metals do, that's hardly an advertisement for supplemental collagen. The virus will still grow and multiply from the supplemental collagen, which will create more virus cells, some of which will feed on heavy metals, and that will result in more neurotoxins in the end anyway. Someone with autoimmune disease, especially an autoimmune condition that involves weakened connective tissue, should not be consuming supplemental collagen. As I say throughout the Medical Medium series, viruses are what create autoimmune disorders. Viruses also create tumors, cysts, nodules, and multiple cancers, including breast cancer and some brain cancers.

As you know well by now, when celery juice is consumed on its own, it breaks down the membranes of viruses and bacteria, weakening the bacterial bodies of bugs like *H. pylori*, *C. difficile*, and strep so it can kill them off. It destroys dangerous varieties of fungus. Celery juice's sodium cluster salts then clean up the mess, neutralizing the pathogenic debris that floats around the body and hinders our own natural collagen. Cluster salts also help neutralize pesticides and herbicides in the body and dislodge toxic heavy metals, uprooting them from organ tissue, such as that in the brain, and bringing the heavy metals closer to the surfaces of organs so that blood vessels can be instrumental in moving the toxic heavy metals out of the body completely. These sodium cluster salts are further responsible for entering the dermis and drawing poison out of the skin, which means drawing the very poisons that threaten to destroy our natural collagen out of our collagen cells.

Cluster salts adhere to the toxins and poisons, neutralizing them and flushing them out of the body. With the technique of pure celery juice on an empty stomach, collagen can then prosper inside your body. New cells can develop—because sodium cluster salts amplify the power of the body to create new protein and collagen cells throughout the body.

The minute you combine supplemental collagen with celery juice in your body, you cancel out celery juice's benefits. Every last sodium cluster salt and enzyme in the juice reacts to the supplemental collagen negatively, as if it were a toxin. As soon as the celery juice–collagen mixture enters your mouth and stomach, the celery juice's cluster salts attach themselves to the foreign collagen and try to rid it from the body via the intestinal tract. Trouble is, collagen's sticky presence engulfs the sodium cluster salts, absorbing them even as the cluster salts are trying to neutralize the supplemental collagen.

There are no benefits to consuming supplemental collagen to begin with, so there are no upsides to be canceled out. There *are* unbelievable benefits to celery juice, and you lose those by mixing it with collagen. The juice's sole purpose becomes trying to carry foreign collagen out through the intestinal tract. The supplemental collagen doesn't even enter the bloodstream; the body eliminates it as waste. Any foreign collagen that does escape the intestinal tract walls gets directed to the liver, giving the organ yet one more troublemaker to sort and stow away. It's somewhat similar to how when we take supplemental ox bile, all the liver gets is the opportunity to clean up a big mess.

The best action we can take is to support our bodies in producing their own collagen (and bile). Taking supplemental collagen doesn't help skin, joints, hair, and nails. For that, you need antioxidants, the proper vitamin B_{12}, and the sulfur that naturally occurs in vegetables, as well as the zinc, magnesium, calcium, and silica found in foods and supplements. Along with drinking your pure celery juice regularly and detoxing the liver of its toxic load, these are the elements that truly support you. As much as you might have heard that supplementing with collagen can help with all of this, know the truth: that's a mistaken theory, one that only ends up taking advantage of consumers.

CELERY TABLETS AND POWDER

Never think you're going to get the same results from celery tablets or powders that you will from fresh celery juice. While some herbs and fruits can benefit you in dried or powdered form, these alternate forms of celery are a waste of money and do not offer anything that celery juice does. Mixing dried celery powder into water is not going to cut it on any level. You can't even reconstitute dehydrated celery juice and expect it to work. For one, its enzymes won't be intact. For another, celery juice's sodium cluster salts work symbiotically with the living water suspended in celery. Cluster salts are actually alive, too. They themselves are a living element of the celery plant—that's

one feature that distinguishes sodium cluster salts from regular salt. Dry them out and they can't serve you in the same way.

Be careful. Don't fall prey to purchasing expensive powders made from celery or celery juice in hopes of mixing them with water and getting the same effect. You can't expect dry or dehydrated celery juice to perform all of the fresh juice's incredible healing tasks. That's like throwing money away.

Also note that celery powder mixes are sometimes used to preserve meat. This leads to a lot of confusion about nitrates and nitrites in celery juice. If these salts have been a worry for you, check out the section on them starting on page 141.

COUMARINS

If you have any concerns about coumarins, you can let them go. Every head of celery has different levels of nutrients and phytochemical compounds. Harvest a planting of celery on one side of the continent, and it can have substantially higher or lower levels of certain compounds than celery from a farm on the other side of the continent. Even from farm to farm and field to field and plant to plant and season to season and day to day, it can vary greatly. Whether it was rainy or not, whether well water was used for irrigation, whether there was enough sun, whether it was colder or hotter, or whether the celery was planted early or late affects what an individual bunch of celery contains versus another, even if they were grown nearby. This is all completely natural.

As far as coumarins go, you'll never pin down an exact ratio of how much is in a 16-ounce glass of celery juice. Coumarins are not toxic to the body. Medical research and science believe that coumarins in other foods may help stimulate white blood cells and defend against cancer. (They haven't examined coumarins in celery juice.) In truth, those health benefits come from various components within a food working together symbiotically, not from coumarins alone. This is how it works with celery juice, too: the entire composition of celery juice is what offers us support. Every single component of a glass of celery juice works symbiotically and synergistically together to help repair and restore a tattered immune system on all levels. This includes reconstructing, replenishing, and rejuvenating the entire white count, including neutrophils, basophils, monocytes, killer cells, and other lymphocytes. While everything celery juice has to offer does this together, among the biggest contributors are the sodium cluster salts destroying viruses so that the viral load drops and the immune system can reestablish itself and improve rapidly. Cluster salts also knock down cancer-causing viruses.

Coumarins specifically repair and restore damaged skin cells in the dermis and have the ability to protect the skin from toxins. They help prevent skin disease, scar tissue, and even skin cancer. Almost all coumarins that we consume head to the skin—a truth that medical research and science have not yet discovered. Since traveling

to other organs is not coumarins' primary pathway, concern that coumarins in celery juice can cause liver damage or even low blood sugar is unfounded. When you drink your 16-ounce glass of celery juice, any coumarins it contains are mainly geared to be delivered to your skin.

DIURETIC EFFECT

Does celery juice have a diuretic effect? An extremely mild one, and it's safe and healthy, so celery juice shouldn't be avoided for this reason. It's nothing like the harsh diuretic effect of coffee, black tea, green tea, or alcohol. I've seen people whose doctors told them to avoid diuretics still consuming green tea because it's believed to be good for health. Celery juice is no more of a diuretic than parsley, spinach, apples, and many other fruits and vegetables that we need for our well-being. The gentle detoxing effect it does have is due to trace minerals—because anything that high in mineral content will encourage your system to flush itself, since trace minerals tend to bind onto toxins.

In celery juice, trace minerals are bundled with sodium cluster salts, and those cluster salts on the whole are what grab on to toxins. When this happens, the body uses its water reserves to flush them, with the cluster salts driving the toxins to the kidneys and bladder for elimination. This is all to your benefit and very different from the way unhealthy diuretics work. If you're still concerned that celery juice is too much of a diuretic for you, try it in very small quantities or chew a celery stick and spit out the pulp to get a little bit in you. While you won't get the benefits that celery juice offers in larger quantities, you will still receive some of celery juice's healing abilities on a smaller, not so easily recognizable scale.

ELIMINATION

If you've heard that celery juice can turn your stools red, don't believe it. Nor can it turn them blue, purple, or yellow. If you consume very large quantities of celery juice, the most it can do is give your stools a slightly green tint. Celery juice can also flush out old, trapped food debris from the intestinal tract. This debris may have subdued tinges of various colors to it, although nothing that would stand out as vibrant or shocking.

FIBER

People sometimes worry that juicing celery and separating it from its fiber means we lose out on the plant's benefits. As we covered in Chapter 4, "How to Make Celery Juice Work for You," juicing celery doesn't strip away vital nutrition. It unlocks it. It is not possible to eat enough celery sticks and chew them to the degree you would have to in order to get what you need from them. That would be very exhausting. And taking chopped celery and throwing it in the best blender there is until it's as smooth as can be is not a way around this. Fiber—which some

sources say is such a loss from celery when it's juiced, and which is still present when you drink blended celery that hasn't been strained—actually gets in the way of celery's ability to help you to its full potential.

Those who are wary of juicing celery are operating under the theory that a whole food is automatically more helpful. Whole-food theories don't apply when we're talking about herbal medicine. Celery's own fiber stops its sodium cluster salts and other components from working. Look at the pharmaceutical and herbalism worlds: they extract compounds from herbs for a reason. To make a medicinal, you're not always looking for the whole plant. Most herbalists will not think it's enough or ideal for most conditions to chew and swallow certain herbs. Just as we do with so many other herbs, we need to extract the medicine hiding in celery—because it's an herb—and that means making celery *juice*. If celery's sodium cluster salts, trace minerals, and enzymes are not extracted from celery's fiber, the fiber keeps them absorbed and basically burns them out.

Careless suggestions and inflexible rules about whole foods taught in nutritional classes and schools have nothing to do with the truth about how you heal chronic symptoms and illness with celery juice. There are no clinical studies to back up the assumption that celery is better for you with its fiber intact. The truth is that with celery, more is better. Not only does juicing celery access potent nutrition; removing fiber also lets you get more celery juice in you, and that's essential for your well-being.

None of which is to put down celery sticks or fiber. Celery itself is great for you. You can still get some (though not all) of the antioxidants, flavonoids, folates, and vitamin C by eating celery, and its fiber does have benefits. Keep celery and fiber in your life. *Also* add celery juice to your life, and enjoy it separately from the whole celery you eat.

GOITROGENS

Goitrogenic compounds are found in some vegetables, herbs, and fruits. Celery is not one of them. (We shouldn't fear goitrogens anyway. The concept has been blown way out of proportion—see *Thyroid Healing* for more.) Any mention of goitrogens, whether in relation to celery juice or otherwise, is a fear tactic that gets in the way of people healing.

HYBRIDIZATION

One misguided theory about celery is that because it's a result of agricultural hybridization, we should be wary of it. Don't let this concern you. Hybrid foods are not genetically modified organisms (GMOs). We've been grafting and hybridizing foods for centuries. And not all varieties are even hybridized; some are heirloom. It's our birthright and our God-given right to use the resources we have growing here and adjust them to fit our needs for survival here on Earth. Hybridization is a natural process; we just help it along so it can provide more for our well-being. Almost every food we

consume is hybridized, and it still holds the nutrition and value that it had long before, when it was in its original source form hundreds or even thousands of years ago.

Hybridized fruits and vegetables such as celery are not acidic or poisonous to the body. Quite the opposite. Celery juice removes acids, breaks down acidosis, restores alkalinity to the body, kills off pathogenic bugs that are poisonous to the body, and removes pesticides, herbicides, and so many other toxic substances from the liver.

If an institution, foundation, group, or panel of influencers in the field of alternative medicine forms a belief system that celery is poisonous to the body, they're making a grave mistake that can hold back healing for billions. Today's standard hybrid versions of organic celery that you find at the store are easy on the body, gentle, alkaline, cleansing, and healing. Heirloom varieties of celery are often too astringent, potent, and abrasive. While they cannot hurt you—they can only help you heal—they're less palatable because they're much more bitter, and therefore you consume less of them. When it comes down to it, the more palatable your celery is, the more of its juice you'll drink and the more benefits you're going to receive.

NITRATES AND NITRITES

Celery and celery juice can't contain any nitrates that are activated or harmful unless the celery has oxidized or been dehydrated. The naturally occurring nitrates in celery don't exist when the celery or fresh celery juice hasn't yet oxidized. When fresh celery juice or celery does oxidize, just as when any herb, vegetable, or fruit oxidizes, then a naturally occurring nitrate can develop. Keep in mind: this naturally occurring nitrate is never harmful in any way, shape, or form and can even be helpful. Celery juice powder and celery powder have oxidized, so they can contain naturally occurring nitrates that developed through the oxidation process. They're not harmful nitrates, though.

These nitrates are not the same variety of nitrates that are considered to be irritating to some people. It's important to know that not all nitrates are the same, just as all people are not the same, all water is not the same, all sugar is not the same, and all protein is not the same. For example, gluten is an entirely different protein from the protein inside meat or the protein inside nuts. Also, the naturally occurring nitrates that can develop in an oxidized form of celery such as celery powder and celery juice powder are not the same as the harmful nitrates that are added to meat and all kinds of other products.

Nitrates are different from nitrites; they're not the same thing. Even celery powder, which does contain naturally occurring nitrates, can't be relied upon as a method for curing foods such as pickles or meat because it still doesn't contain nitrites. Fresh celery juice also doesn't contain nitrites. Nothing naturally occurring in celery and celery juice is harmful. This is the same for pure celery powder and pure celery juice powder. Here's where

the confusion lies: harmful nitrates can be added to celery powder, celery juice powder, or celery salt by a company that makes it or uses it to make another product. Celery gets false blame for harmful nitrates in preserved meats and other products—when the truth is that it's a classic case of contaminating celery with add-ins. Your fresh celery juice cannot have harmful nitrates in it unless you add them yourself.

If you don't drink fresh celery juice because you believe it contains harmful nitrates or nitrites, then you are going to lose the unique healing opportunity that fresh celery juice—which does not contain nitrates or nitrites—can provide.

OXALATES

Do not be concerned about oxalate (oxalic acid) in celery juice. The myth that certain leafy green vegetables and herbs such as celery are high in oxalates and therefore harmful is completely misguided. This myth prevents so many people from getting the powerful and needed nutrients and healing properties that foods deemed high in oxalates could provide to them.

Oxalates are not the concern they are believed to be. There are oxalates in every single fruit and vegetable on the planet. Oxalates are entirely different from food to food—the oxalates in a plum, for example, are much different from those in a piece of cheese. This is an underfunded area of medical research and science, so medical communities don't truly know how different forms of oxalate react, relate to, or accumulate in the body. Claims that oxalates should make us fear celery juice are unproven and unsubstantiated. In reality, these foods do not cause us any harm. Rather, they provide us with critical healing phytochemicals, vitamins, minerals, and more.

The vast array of nutrients in so-called high-oxalate leafy greens and celery are some of the most beneficial available to us. Medical research and science have not yet discovered that fruits, vegetables, leafy greens, and herbs contain anti-oxalates that prevent oxalates from causing the damage that current trends tell us they cause. Oxalates are widespread, whether we like it or not. So are antidotes to oxalates. If there's any food that counters what we fear oxalates do, it's celery juice. The common belief is that foods high in oxalates produce kidney stones and gallstones. If celery juice were really a concern here, how would it be that it helps *dissolve* kidney stones and gallstones? It's not oxalates that cause trouble with uric acid in the kidneys. It's proteins that create kidney stones and gout by bogging down the liver.

People also fear spinach because of oxalate rumors. I've been witness to decades of spinach bringing people back to vitality, rejuvenating them, and helping them recover from chronic symptoms and illness. Raw spinach is even safer for this than cooked and is extremely healthy. Don't toss out valuable healing tools like spinach and celery juice due to mistaken theories.

PSORALENS

Psoralens will constitute another fear tactic used to deter people from consuming celery. These phytochemical compounds, which reside in almost all fruits, vegetables, and herbs, are helpful for the immune system and for healing our bodies. Any psoralens present in celery are harmless. They do not create sun sensitivities or dermatitis. Instead, celery juice's psoralens help rid people of these and other skin conditions, as you saw in Chapter 3.

SALICYLIC ACID

Salicylic acid, also known as salicylate, is another myth used as a fear tactic that deters people from experiencing the healing benefits of celery juice. The theory that individuals are sensitive to salicylic acid from fruits and vegetables has not been proven by medical research and science. Since celery is not a vegetable, it shouldn't be grouped in this theory anyway. Celery juice is an herbal medicine that helps reverse food chemical compound sensitivities that many people develop from gluten, dairy, corn, eggs, and soy. The medicinal compounds in celery juice rid the body of toxins, viruses, and bacteria, which are mostly responsible for food sensitivities in the first place.

SODIUM

As we've explored, the sodium in celery is not the same as the sodium in food products or even in high-quality Celtic sea salt or Himalayan rock salt. We're not a low-salt society. We're inundated with salt in daily life. While there are people who are mindful about it, they're in the minority. The majority of restaurants worldwide rely on salt. If you had never in your life eaten food with added salt and then went out to eat or tried a packaged snack, you would be staggered by the overpowering nature of all the salt we put in food. We're a "salted" culture right now.

Where does all that salt you eat go? Does it just flow right out of your body as easily as it entered? No. Even the most premium salt from a jar of organic salsa or the healthiest dehydrated crackers or salted nut mix stores itself deep inside cells, deep inside organs, and crystallizes there. Salt particularly embeds itself in your liver, because your liver tries to gather it up from your bloodstream to protect you from falling ill from overuse of salt, which is a part of nearly everybody's everyday life. There in the liver, salt sticks around for years and becomes toxic if we're not cleansing it. Someone who's worried about the sodium in celery should instead be worried about the onslaught of salt in packaged foods, restaurant dishes, and even home cooking.

The sodium in celery juice is a reprieve from all that. It provides sodium that not only doesn't harm us, it helps us. When people are concerned about celery juice and sodium, they're really saying they don't understand celery. It's a blind assumption with no research or science to back it up. In truth, the sodium in celery juice helps loosen up and break apart toxic sodium crystal deposits in the liver and elsewhere in the body—because the sodium in celery is different. Celery juice's sodium cluster salts drive toxic sodium deposits out of the body by attaching themselves to the toxic sodium and carrying it away. Further, the sodium in celery juice is what our blood needs and can use the most. Neurotransmitters thrive on this variety of sodium, which has just the right minerals and trace minerals attached.

Remember from Chapter 2: rather than containing neurotransmitter chemical building blocks in the form of partial electrolytes as other foods do—minerals that find their way to neurons by chance, depending on what someone is eating and drinking—celery juice is the only food on the planet to offer complete, activated, and living electrolytes. Even coconut water, a great natural source of electrolytes, only offers pieces of them. The same goes for man-made electrolyte products: manufacturers add minerals based on what nutritional science merely theorizes will help comprise usable electrolytes. These products aren't even marketed to help neurons. Instead we hear generally, "It's good for the body" and "We need electrolytes." Celery juice doesn't only help build neurotransmitter chemicals piecemeal to support neurons; it offers complete neurotransmitter chemicals that are already bonded together to reignite weakened neurotransmitters and offer the ultimate neuron relief. When electricity flows, it can flow freely. Celery juice's naturally occurring beneficial sodium is an integral part of that.

As I say, all water is not the same, and all sugar is not the same. Well, add this to the list: all salt is not the same.

WATER

On the subject of water, if anyone tells you that drinking celery juice is the same as drinking water, know this: they are far from the same. Water does have naturally occurring electrolytes, especially if it's high-quality water. Still, those electrolytes provide entirely different benefits from those in celery juice. This is not even like comparing apples to oranges; it's like apples to beef. Water and celery juice are two completely different substances. Only the herb celery contains the sodium cluster salts, special enzymes, and particular trace minerals that make celery juice what it is.

As for putting a pinch of salt in a glass of water and thinking that's the same or better, this is even more misguided. If you exercise and sweat a lot and a trainer, guru, or health professional tells you to put salt in your water to get hydrated again, all you're doing is dehydrating yourself further. Adding salt to water is dehydrating on a deep level. Celery juice is *hydrating* on a deep level. What you really need after workouts is celery juice (plus a calorie source—refer back to "Timing Tips" in Chapter 4). Not to mention that even the highest-quality Himalayan rock salt or sea salt is still not on a par with the beneficial sodium in celery. Celery juice and salted water are two different worlds. Which world are you living in?

By the way, I'll say it again: mixing celery juice with water is not a good move—because they're so different, they clash. There's a friction between them. Adding water to celery juice dilutes the sodium cluster salts and deactivates them while also interfering with the trace minerals and enzymes, some of the most powerful aspects of celery juice that help us heal. Adding ice cubes to celery juice has the same effect. While combining water and celery juice won't hurt you, it's not productive: it doesn't enhance celery juice on any level, and in truth it destroys the ability of celery juice to heal the body. That's right: it interferes with all the nutrients in celery juice, from basic ones such as its vitamin K to its unique variety of vitamin C, disrupting the delivery of these nutrients to the body and completely stopping celery juice from offering anything.

Here's another point to keep in mind when it comes to water and celery juice: some sources say that people only feel better from celery juice because they're getting hydrated by its water content. These sources say that it has little or nothing to do with the celery juice itself. This is an inadvertent insult to the chronically ill. It's like telling people who have been sick for months or years, who have looked for healing in so many different ways, that they never thought to drink more water. Staying hydrated is the first piece of advice that many people get regarding any aspect of health and wellness. This advice comes from magazines, health coaches, and doctors alike, and those who are suffering listen. They carry their water bottles everywhere and become committed to drinking water morning, noon, and night.

When sources say that the only reason the chronically ill are getting their lives back from celery juice is because it offers water, it's almost inconceivable. It shows confusion and a lack of experience and understanding of what people with chronic symptoms and illnesses must do on a daily basis to survive. Yes, celery juice has more water content than many other sources, and yes, its hydro-bioactive water is beneficial. It's not a simple matter of water content that's getting people better, though. If it were, everyone who had tried increasing their water intake would have already gotten better. They would have gotten better, too, from paying attention to FODMAPs (fermentable oligosaccharides, disaccharides, monosaccharides, and polyols) and scrambling to test every other sort of diet under the sun. (By the way, celery juice will help an individual reverse a FODMAP intolerance by helping restore the liver and intestinal tract.) They would have gotten better from the dozens of doctors they visited—ranging from conventional to functional to alternative—and the tens or hundreds of thousands of dollars they spent in pursuit of answers.

When these people turn to celery juice and find results, it's not the first time they've paid attention to what they put in their bodies and simply a sign that they've started taking better care of themselves. These are people who have been in the weeds, tried everything there is. When they finally bring in celery juice, they find that it's the first thing that actually starts turning their life around. These individuals deserve more respect than hearing that their healing is only thanks to water.

FUTURE FEAR TACTICS

The rumors we've just looked at are relatively minor. Get ready. Because of the immense healing that celery juice is doing globally, I foresee a bigger attack on celery juice someday, one that far surpasses the hundreds of smaller forms of doubt and denial from various sources that say it's not doing anything for anyone. When a force is healing people on a global level to this degree—reducing hospitalizations and helping people recover more quickly from the flu, food poisoning, mental illness, and chronic symptoms and conditions that require pharmaceuticals—and when medical research and science don't have it contained and industries don't have a way to make money off it, it can invite attempts at sabotage.

When will this bigger attack come? Who will initiate it? I don't know. That comes down to free will. I know that the ambush is on its way. This attempt at undermining celery juice's power could come in many forms. The first booby trap has already been set as a small-scale rumor that too much celery juice is bad. By the time this book is published, an authority or industry might have stepped up to perpetuate the idea that people should instead limit themselves to a stalk or so a day, either as a few celery sticks with peanut butter or juiced with a whole bunch of vegetables. (That peanut butter recommendation, by the way, will only support the high-fat trend, and if you want to know why that's not helping anyone, check out *Liver Rescue*.) It's even likely that a document will be released claiming a study was performed, and that this document will warn people off celery juice, with no one realizing that the whole endeavor was funded solely to produce great concern.

Another tactic that will snare many well-meaning people is the anecdotal evidence confusion that we addressed at the end of Chapter 6, "Healing and Detox Answers." What sounds like a voice of reason saying that people's healing needs to go under a microscope to gain validity and credibility is likely to get louder and louder. This will come across as a protective message, all logic, and it will be crafted to make the celery juice movement appear foolish and out of touch with the rigors of scientific inquiry. It will effectively put the concept of healing in a box and say that getting better from celery juice doesn't fit in that box and therefore isn't real. Wrapped up in this will be placebo confusion—claims that any benefits felt from celery juice are nothing more than the placebo effect. If this were true, the placebo effect would have healed people's problems years ago, when they tried any number of techniques or diets in what must have felt like an endless search for health. Rather than humbling themselves to the ever greater numbers of people getting their lives back from celery juice, sources that lean on "anecdotal" and "placebo"—however well-meaning these sources are in their devotion to the medical establishment—will cast doubt on countless people's authentic recovery. This will be a regression that takes us back to the state of mind that dominated in the 1950s through

1990s, when people struggling with chronic illness had to try so hard to convince their doctors and sometimes family members that they were really sick, when they were too often doubted only because the medical industry was slow at diagnosing or finding causes for chronic health problems. This regression in the way chronically ill people are treated will help no one.

Later on, it could be an interest group with funding behind it that tries to create fear around an invented problem with celery juice. It could be regulatory issues around growing celery—elevated fees for celery farms that produce high yields, forcing farmers to grow other crops so they can make ends meet. It could be a fabricated contamination scare. Even if celery itself has not yielded one issue, any whispered rumor that's put out there to incite fear could catch on like wildfire. Or there could be an attack on celery seed, whether in the form of a mandated ration on seed supply or the creation of GMO celery seeds to put out in the world to interfere with uncontaminated celery. In whatever form it's going to arrive, at whatever time, mark my words: the unjust attack is coming.

I say all this to prepare you, not to worry you. If you're prepared, you can stay strong. When messaging is purposely put out to try to scare you away from consuming celery juice, stand firm. Think about the history, already going back decades, of what celery juice has done for people's healing progress. Look to the history that's building in the moment. There are people alive today who are positive they wouldn't be alive if not for the celery juice movement. Weigh that against the fearmongering.

Because celery juice is not a trend, it can't burn out. Nor will it float into the abyss of "Does anybody really know if this works?" where many health trends eventually vanish. (Most trends that don't vanish are given a heartbeat by the continual funding of investors trying to breathe new life into them.) No matter what tactics try to undermine your trust in celery juice, remember: celery juice works. That's plain to see. Don't let anything shake your confidence in the healing you've experienced from celery juice. When the rumors keep coming as the years go by, learn to laugh them off and feel sorry for those who perpetuate them. They don't realize that their own fear or skepticism or sense of competition will only keep them from experiencing a healing miracle of our time.

The naysayers issuing hot takes on celery juice's silliness don't realize they're time stamping themselves. Nor are the sources that perpetuate misinformation about celery juice aware that they're not positioning themselves as savvily as they think they are. They don't realize that by publicly writing off celery juice—not realizing that celery is an herb, for example, and saying that no

vegetable can be this beneficial—they're locking themselves into an already dated viewpoint. They're historically documenting their skepticism of a healing movement that is showing itself to be larger than life. The doubt should have come in 2015, when my first book, *Medical Medium*, was published featuring a section on celery juice. Years later, now that celery juice has caught on at a global scale, it's a little late to say it doesn't work. Attempts to discredit celery juice, even as some of those attempts catch on for a time, will only get more and more dated.

If celery juice doubt gets you riled up, keep this in mind: when someone takes issue with celery juice, what they're really communicating is how lost they are. In their hearts, if they stopped to consider it, there is no way they would want to discredit people who, after months or years of suffering, are able to get out of bed, care for their children, or go back to earning a living again thanks to celery juice. The naysayers are not compassionless. They're simply searching, and on that search for the truth of life, they're lost. You are found—you have found the truth of celery juice, and the truth of celery juice has found you. With that truth, you can show other searchers the way.

CHAPTER 8

More Healing Guidance

Celery juice can help heal so many issues quickly. It also exists outside of food belief systems. It's immune to food belief systems. It's above food belief systems. One of the many reasons for this is that celery is an herb, and celery juice is an herbal medicine. No matter what diet you subscribe to, you can apply celery juice.

That said, I'm the first to tell you that celery juice alone is not the be-all and end-all for many people. It can be, for the person with a symptom such as mild acid reflux. With celery juice, someone's heartburn could be gone for good. In other cases, the be-all and end-all is celery juice *as part of a team* of healing protocols. As mighty and powerful as celery juice is, it is one tool among many that I recommend.

It can get confusing out there. Once the Medical Medium community started spreading the word about celery juice, its popularity was noticed by influencers who had never even heard of these books. Celery juice has been used to build platforms without pointing to its origin—an origin that

offers other critical information for restoring the health of the chronically ill. Celery juice has been used to get clicks. Sometimes this is a disheartening move made without remembering compassion for the people who are sick. Sometimes it's only that an influencer is excited about celery juice, which I celebrate, and doesn't realize that they're leaving out some critical pieces. Either way, this runaway popularity means that the tag "celery juice," accompanied by vibrant green photos, has made its way through the world independent of the other healing information meant to go along with it.

That's where the confusion lies. Someone who's struggling with SIBO, for example, and starts drinking celery juice because she saw a popular post online could find that her gut problems don't heal as fast as she wants. That's because the source that recommended celery juice never directed her to the proper, supportive dietary guidelines—or that source even made misguided suggestions, such as eating lots of eggs, which fed the bacterial overgrowth and actively stymied her healing. These sorts of contradictions dilute the message of celery juice. They can make people who try celery juice feel like they've been there, done that, and it's just another unfulfilled promise—because at the same time they're bringing celery juice into their lives, they're also following guidance to consume liberal amounts of items like bone broth, grass-fed butter, and coffee, and that holds back healing. Yes, even with items in the diet that could be feeding the bacteria behind SIBO or the virus behind another condition, if they keep going with celery juice they can at least prevent the condition from worsening, or they can experience improvements in other areas of their health. It's not all or nothing. If celery juice isn't doing everything you want it to, though, don't give up on it. Turn to these ways to make it do even better. A mom who's struggling to pay her bills, hold down her career, or take care of her children while living with a new diagnosis of ME/CFS, MS, or Lyme disease may lose five years of her life because she quit celery juice. If only she'd been told the right foods to avoid, the right recipes to lean on, the right supplements to incorporate, and the right trends to avoid so that celery juice could have shown its worth to her.

If you're looking for better results than what you get from only celery juice, you can apply it to your life along with additional healing guidance from the Medical Medium series. That's what so many readers before you have done to get to a better place. Those with more serious, chronic conditions typically need both. Because this information comes from the same source as celery juice, it all works together to bring you more advanced recovery. I applaud anyone who has the courage to recognize the source of celery juice. I applaud anyone who has the guts to stand up for chronic illness sufferers and recognize the other healing guidance from that same source.

Knowing what's behind your health struggles is a helpful component of moving forward, which is why I addressed symptom and illness causes in Chapter 3 (and throughout the Medical Medium series). When people don't know that a virus or other hidden cause is the reason for their suffering, and they don't know what fuels or vanquishes that hidden cause, they often give up on celery juice too soon. That means they lose a golden opportunity.

DIETARY TIPS

When someone says, "I've got to clean up my diet," what does that really mean? There are so many definitions of healthy eating these days that it can feel impossible to figure out the best foods to put on your plate and leave off it. There are some obvious answers: try to avoid fried foods and rich desserts, and eat more vegetables and leafy greens. What about fruit? It's a controversial topic. The truth is: don't fear it. Its nutrients are critical for healing. (If that doesn't give you permission enough to eat fruit, check out the "Fruit Fear" chapter of *Medical Medium*.)

No matter your food belief system, here's a tip to support celery juice's work in your body: lower the amount of dietary fat you consume by about 50 percent while bringing in more of what I call *critical clean carbohydrates* to fill up on instead. CCC include fresh fruit, potatoes, sweet potatoes, winter squash, and even oatmeal.

If you eat a plant-based diet, lowering your fat consumption means reducing the amount of nuts, seeds, peanut butter, other nut butters, oils, avocados, coconut, and olives you eat. If your diet is more focused on animal products, try to eat less beef (even if grass fed), chicken, turkey, and fish while also reducing plant fats. Try to avoid dairy, pork, and eggs entirely (more in a moment). Whichever side of the aisle you're on, try to cut your fat consumption in half by only having fats once a day, for example, instead of two or three times daily, or waiting until lunchtime or later to eat fats. Again, in their absence, bring in more CCC as filling nourishment. Also bring in more leafy greens such as spinach, mâche, butter leaf and other lettuces, lettuce mixes, arugula, dandelion greens, mustard greens, and kale.

These steps are vital when you want celery juice's herbal properties to work even better at reducing your symptoms or conditions and improving your health. They're also just a few recommendations that come from the Medical Medium series. You'll sometimes hear people refer to "the Medical Medium protocol." The truth is that there is no one protocol. There are a variety of protocols that you can tailor to yourself,

using your own expertise about your health situation to guide you about which to choose. For a more advanced understanding of how (and why) to eat for your particular health issue, look into the other Medical Medium books.

HEAVY METAL DETOX

Toxic heavy metals are a large part of why we're struggling with illness in the world today. It's imperative that we take the opportunity to remove these heavy metals—including mercury, aluminum, copper, lead, cadmium, and nickel—from our bodies, most importantly from our brains and livers. The Heavy Metal Detox Smoothie accompanies celery juice in this mission very effectively, providing even more support for celery juice to do its job in the healing process.

(Not that you should drink the smoothie at the same time as celery juice—as always, you want to enjoy your celery juice apart from other food and drink. As we covered in Chapter 5, "The Celery Juice Cleanse," the smoothie makes an excellent breakfast 15 to 30 minutes following your celery juice.)

This Heavy Metal Detox Smoothie recipe was not created yesterday. It has been in use for many years within the Medical Medium community, and it has a powerful history of working. It is a big piece of how people find healing—it has a record of helping reverse illness and turn lives around. The smoothie's ingredients work together safely and uniquely to remove toxic heavy metals from organs and deliver them out of your body. That's unlike other heavy metal detox modalities that have been in use over the years, methods that sloppily pick up and then let go of metals as they're carried through your system—which only ends up shifting toxic heavy metals around in your body and creating additional problems. The Heavy Metal Detox Smoothie's five key ingredients of wild blueberries, cilantro, barley grass juice powder, spirulina, and Atlantic dulse function as a team, dislodging, extracting, and then responsibly carrying toxic heavy metals all the way out of your body. You'll find more on this detox teamwork in *Medical Medium* and *Thyroid Healing*.

And now for the recipe, so you can join the growing number of people who have discovered the power of the Heavy Metal Detox Smoothie:

HEAVY METAL DETOX SMOOTHIE RECIPE

Makes 1 serving

What you'll need:

2 bananas

2 cups wild blueberries

1 cup cilantro

1 teaspoon barley grass juice powder

1 teaspoon spirulina

1 tablespoon Atlantic dulse

1 orange

1 cup water

Combine the bananas, blueberries, cilantro, barley grass juice powder, spirulina, and dulse with the juice of one orange in a high-speed blender and blend until smooth. Add up to 1 cup of water if a thinner consistency is desired. Serve and enjoy!

UNPRODUCTIVE FOODS

There are some foods that it's a good idea to avoid altogether if you want optimal healing. This has nothing to do with a belief system about "good" and "bad" foods. It is simply because some of these foods feed viruses and bacteria. Further, these foods interfere with celery juice working as well as it can for you. If you can't live without these foods, you're still allowed to drink celery juice without making these changes. Or try avoiding just one or two of them, and see how it goes from there. You will still get to experience improvements in your health. If you're looking for major improvements, on the other hand, try skipping all of these foods and ingredients to get celery juice to work even better for you. By avoiding them, you minimize disruptions to celery juice's critically healing phytochemical compounds.

- Eggs
- Dairy (including milk, cheese, butter, cream, yogurt, kefir, ghee, whey protein)
- Gluten
- Vinegar (including apple cider vinegar—ACV)
- Nutritional yeast
- Fermented foods
- Soy
- Corn
- Pork products (including bacon, sausage, ham)
- Canola oil
- Natural flavors

HERBS AND SUPPLEMENTS

Trying herbal supplements is an optional step beyond all the dietary advice above. You don't have to play in Supplement Land if you don't want to—drinking celery juice, lowering fats, and adding in healing CCC and leafy greens will help address all your problems. Supplements are for people looking for something more because their situations are perplexing to them and their doctors. You'll find a treasure trove of supplement options for specific symptoms and conditions in *Medical Medium*, *Thyroid Healing*, and *Liver Rescue*.

I'm continually asked: What is the most effective form of a given supplement, and does it really matter? Yes, it matters greatly. There are subtle and sometimes critical differences among the various supplement types available that can affect how quickly your viral or bacterial load dies off, if at all; whether your central nervous system repairs itself and how fast; how quickly your inflammation reduces; and how long it takes for your symptoms and conditions to heal. The supplement variety you choose can make or break your progress. For example, many herbal tinctures contain alcohol, which interferes with an herb's phytochemical compounds, feeds pathogens such as the Epstein-Barr virus and all forms of unproductive bacteria, and kills off good bacteria in the intestinal tract. To speed up healing, you need the right kinds of supplements. For these very important reasons, I offer a directory on my website (www.medicalmedium.com) of the best forms of each supplement I recommend. If you want the best barley grass juice powder, spirulina, or vitamin C on the market, for example, you'll find it in the directory.

SODIUM CLUSTER SALT SUPPORT

A clean, healthy gut and a clean, healthy liver allow celery juice's sodium cluster salts to travel most effectively to the brain, skin, and other far reaches of the body. How do you get a clean, healthy gut and liver? With long-term use of celery juice and other Medical Medium protocols combined. They all serve one another. This is one reason why people who have used the teachings in this series to spruce up their diets by reducing fats and increasing fruits, potatoes, sweet potatoes, winter squash, and leafy greens will often find that celery juice starts working even better for them: the dietary shift helped reduce pathogens, mucus, rancid fats, and toxins in the liver and gut—and that cleared the way for celery juice do its job better. In turn, these people keep feeling better.

On the other hand, people who tend to reach for mainstream "healthy" options like butter stirred into coffee, protein shakes, and eggs can unknowingly feed viruses

including shingles, EBV, cytomegalovirus, and HHV-6 that are hiding out in the liver and elsewhere. This is also why some people with a very toxic liver—which leads to a thickened, dirty bloodstream with lots of fat in it as well as lots of old, rotting debris, rancid fat, and loads of bacteria in the intestinal tract—who try celery juice for the first time may feel it's a bit of a shock to the system. Celery juice induces a rapid healing response as its sodium cluster salts kill off unproductive bacteria, yeast, toxic funguses, and viruses, and that can lead to a quick bout of diarrhea. At the same time, celery juice is properly dissolving rancid fats that are lining the intestinal tract, and that can cause a bit of acid reflux, because it's the most powerfully healing apparatus that a person has consumed yet.

As celery juice starts to do its work, if someone is helping it along with dietary shifts too, then the liver keeps getting cleaner and starts to come out of stagnancy, the intestinal linings get scrubbed, the pathogenic load of viruses and bacteria is reduced, and blood is no longer thick and toxic with fats and poisons. And if someone is using the Heavy Metal Detox Smoothie, too, the elevation of toxic heavy metals in the system is reduced. Someone who reaches this state of healing is now in the position where sodium cluster salts can do their job best.

One critical mission of sodium cluster salts is to bind onto and deliver nutrients to the brain and other parts of the body. We have to see cluster salts as a caravan dropping people off along the way. Only instead of people, the cluster salt caravan can transport and deliver a variety of minerals, other nutrients, and chemical compounds from foods. If you don't have ample glucose in your bloodstream, though, you miss out. This is part of why it's so important to have CCC in your diet. Fruit, winter squash, potatoes, and sweet potatoes give you high-quality glucose—and that glucose binds onto the chemical compounds such as sodium cluster salts from celery, driving whole sodium cluster salt caravans of nutrients deep into tissue and cells in the body, including into deep internal organs.

A high-fat diet isn't beneficial when it comes to accessing this powerful healing mechanism that celery juice offers. If you're on a ketogenic or otherwise low-carb diet, it means you're running on fat calories, and your glucose reserves are diminishing. You lose the opportunity, then, for glucose to drive cluster salts where they're needed—and for glucose to be the key that opens the doors to let sodium cluster salt caravans deliver nutrients throughout the body. The good news is that most keto diets now incorporate sugars, even though nobody realizes it. Thank goodness that avocado has a good portion of natural sugars, as do the nuts and seeds allowed in many keto diets. While this renders the diets not technically ketogenic,

it means that individuals can better access what celery juice has to offer. Whatever type of diet or non-diet you follow, reducing fats will help all of this work better.

A sodium cluster salt caravan tends to drop nutrients off quickly, leaving them in the liver or bloodstream. Certain amino acids and minerals have more staying power and can hitch a ride with cluster salts all the way to the brain. We don't always get these amino acids and minerals in our diets, though, especially if we're eating less-than-healthy concoctions of foods. It's another reason why it's in our best interest not to limit the healing steps we take in our lives to drinking celery juice. If we're also being mindful to incorporate a variety of fruits, other CCC, vegetables, leafy greens, and herbs into our diets in general, then we're providing celery juice's cluster salts with more nutrients to deliver to brain tissue (and other organs)—and this can greatly improve a variety of conditions. Neurotransmitter chemicals can be enhanced. The rate at which brain cells die off can be reduced.

If we let them, sodium cluster salts become a critical part of our existence. They are their own universe of life that bonds to our own life, helping sustain us here on Earth for the long term.

"Celery juice is simple and it's real and it works, with only good intentions behind it, and that threatens to expose other popular health 'remedies' as being not so pure, effective, or aboveboard."

— Anthony William, Medical Medium

CHAPTER 9

Alternatives to Celery Juice

What to do if you can't find celery or celery juice, or if you can't have celery? Step one: don't panic. It happens. With so many people making celery juice now, it's become a fairly normal occurrence for stores to run out of celery due to high demand. Sometimes, too, farms are in between plantings or can't grow enough to keep up with orders. Sometimes tough weather threatens crops. We can't take it out on our growers or grocers, and we can't despair about our health, either. Instead, step two: turn to an alternative. The recipes in this chapter will get you through when you can't access celery juice.

If the reason you can't make your celery juice is that you're traveling without a juicer, see if you can seek out a nearby fresh juice spot before you turn to these backup options. You may find that a local natural foods store will make it for you. If that doesn't work, maybe you can at least pick up some celery sticks, or bring some with you, and chew on those. While they're not going to do what celery juice does, they will at least keep your body emotionally and

spiritually connected to the celery plant while helping your cells recall the experience of celery juice. It's a way of letting your body know that you haven't quit, that you're only traveling right now. If you're feeling really committed, you can even go so far as to chew the celery and then spit out the pulp.

As we explored in Chapter 4, it may be that you have an allergic reaction to celery, so celery juice is not an option for you at all. In that case, select one of these recipes as your mainstay and commit to it as though it were celery juice. It will still bring you many healing benefits, and over time you may even find that healing your body alleviates your celery allergy.

When you can't have or get celery juice for whatever reason and that has you turning to one of these alternatives instead, it's a good idea to refer to other Medical Medium healing information at the same time. If after reading the previous chapter you're still hungry for details, look into the other books in the series. There, you can find the foods, further dietary guidance, supplements, recipes, and even meditations that speak to you to give your body extra support in the absence of celery juice.

As you look at the recipes below, know that your first choice as a staple in place of celery juice is pure cucumber juice. The same guideline applies: pure cucumber juice, not cucumber-apple juice or cucumber-kale juice, as delicious as those would be at other times of day, and not cucumber juice with ACV added or ice cubes floating in it. Cucumber juice on its own is key. If cucumbers or cucumber juice are not accessible, then select one of the alternative options.

CUCUMBER JUICE RECIPE

Makes 1 serving

Cucumber juice follows the same principle as celery juice: keep it simple. In order to make 16 ounces of cucumber juice (1 adult serving), here's what you'll need:

What you'll need:

2 large cucumbers

How to make it:

Rinse the cucumbers and run them through the juicer of your choice. Drink immediately, on an empty stomach, for best results.

If you don't have access to a juicer, here's how you can make it instead:

Rinse the cucumbers, chop them, and blend them in a high-speed blender until smooth. Strain well (a nut milk bag is handy for this). Drink immediately, on an empty stomach, for best results.

GINGER WATER RECIPE

Makes 1 serving

What you'll need:

1 to 2 inches fresh ginger

½ lemon (optional)

2 cups (16 ounces) water

2 teaspoons raw honey (optional)

How to make it:

Grate the ginger into the water and add the juice from half of a freshly cut lemon if desired. (Alternatively, you can chop the ginger into a few small pieces and squeeze them in a garlic press. Be sure to remove the pulp from the press afterward, chop it finely, and add it to the water, too.)

Allow the water to steep for at least 15 minutes, ideally longer. (You can even leave it steeping in the fridge overnight.)

Strain the water. Add raw honey if desired and enjoy warm, cold, or room temperature on an empty stomach.

TIP

- As an alternative to grating the ginger, try chopping it into a few small pieces and squeezing them in a garlic press—it will act like a mini juicer. Be sure to take out the "pulp" from the press afterward, chop it finely, and add it to the water, too.

ALOE WATER RECIPE

Makes 1 serving

What you'll need:

2-inch piece of fresh aloe leaf

2 cups (16 ounces) water

How to make it:

This recipe is based on using a large, store-bought aloe leaf, which you can find in the produce section of many grocery stores. If you're using a homegrown aloe plant, it will likely have smaller, skinnier leaves, so cut off more. Either way, avoid using the bitter base of the leaf.

Carefully slice your section of aloe leaf open, filleting it as if it were a fish and trimming away the green skin and spikes. Scoop out the clear gel and place it in the blender.

Add the water to the blender and blend for 10 to 20 seconds, until the aloe is thoroughly liquefied. Drink immediately, on an empty stomach, for best results.

TIPS

- Fresh aloe leaves can be found in the produce section of many supermarkets.
- Save the remainder of the aloe leaf by wrapping the cut end in a damp towel or plastic wrap and storing in the refrigerator for up to 2 weeks.

LEMON OR LIME WATER RECIPE

What you'll need:

½ lemon or lime

2 cups (16 ounces) water

How to make it:

Squeeze the juice from half of a freshly cut lemon or lime into the water. Enjoy on an empty stomach.

TIP

- Lemons and limes travel well. When you're on the road and missing your kitchen, make sure to pack a few lemons and limes so you can enjoy this fresh tonic when you're far from home.

"Regardless of what they're told by those who have never struggled with sickness, people are getting better. Regardless of what they're told by the lost souls who don't understand, millions of people are healing, gaining control over their lives, and witnessing miracles. They're discovering that it is not a dream. It's real."

— Anthony William, Medical Medium

CHAPTER 10

A Healing Movement

What if millions of people had been stuck with symptoms and illnesses for months, years, or even decades? What if they had tried everything—switching diets, altering lifestyles, getting rid of processed foods, taking heaps of supplements, visiting countless doctors—and after all that, they still hadn't moved the needle with their health? And what if, after being sick for so long and struggling so hard to heal, they finally found an answer that worked? Wouldn't that be incredible? An answer that pulled them out of the darkness. An answer that, for the first time, brought them into the light.

What if they found themselves able to function again, in less pain, able to go about their day, able to get their lives back? What if they were able to feel like they once did— or even better—and they found hope for the future again, now that they had discovered something that actually worked and continued to work each day and didn't just fade away? We're not talking one person out of every hundred feeling a little better one day out of every month. We're talking about thousands building to hundreds of thousands building to millions recovering, as if it were a dream come true.

Wouldn't it be amazing? Or would we believe them? Would we think they had exaggerated their healing? Would we doubt that they had ever been that sick to begin with? Would we find it literally incredible, not to be believed? Well, we can ask ourselves that question honestly, because there *are* millions—really, billions—of people who are sick and unable to move forward and have tried everything and can't find the answers. That's not a dystopian vision of a bleak future; that's where we are today. And at last, increasing numbers of these people are getting better.

Regardless of what they're told by those who have never struggled with sickness, people are getting better. Regardless of what they're told by those who don't know what it's like to be knocked down by a health challenge, who don't know what it takes to get through the day while suffering in physical and emotional pain, and yet who still want to be influencers in the field of health while inadvertently spreading misinformation, people are getting better with celery juice. Regardless of what they're told by the lost souls who don't understand, millions of people are healing, gaining control over their lives, and witnessing miracles. They're discovering that it is not a dream. It's real.

Whether we like it or not, whether we wish it would go away or we think it's wonderful, the healing movement that you've read about in this book is happening, and it's not going to stop. It's a movement that offers us the rare opportunity to rise out of the ashes of sickness and heal. It's bigger than any of us now.

You can choose to ignore it, and I absolutely respect that. You have every right. You can also accept it and use it to heal yourself and others around you and in the process become a believer. Or you could even choose the middle ground: give it a try for yourself, to get yourself healthier and protect yourself and keep yourself healthy for years to come, and decide not to shout all this from the rooftops. Whichever approach you choose, there will be millions who believe—and more than believe, they know. Their knowledge is enough to hold a candle for you.

They know because they couldn't get out of bed before. They couldn't see clearly. They couldn't hear well. As great as their pain was, they were also numb from being trapped in chronic illness, too often unseen and unheard. And then they started to heal, and they kept healing. Their faith is so bright because it truly worked for them, and it's still working, and they're no longer stuck, hopeless, with no answers. Not only are they no longer hopeless, they're past having hope. They don't have to hope anymore that something will come along to save them. It came along, they grabbed hold of it, and they saved themselves. They went from hopeless to "I hope this works" to "It has helped. It has worked. I am getting better. I am getting my life back."

I remember early in my life offering straight celery juice to the many who needed it because they were struggling and even suffering with symptoms and illnesses. I remember watching them recover, gain strength, and heal. I remember thinking, *If something really works, it will stand the test of time.* It made perfect logical sense that if celery juice was working and people were healing, the world had to know about it and it would catch on over time.

And miraculously, the world does know about it now. Not because a massive campaign of endless money and media created it. The movement came from another source entirely: the voice of each individual who adopted this healing miracle, who stayed with it and passed it along to others they met along the way. It was a quiet movement for a long time, one that grew naturally and organically. Not only did the movement have a soul to it, it had a truth to it, and it became strong before most everyone knew about it. And when the time was right, it became so strong that it swelled into a tidal wave, with masses of people ready to speak the truth about the healing they had experienced. The wave hit shore and flowed over the earth practically all at once. People who hadn't paid attention before shook their heads, whether in amazement, bafflement, or disbelief. "Where did this come from?" they asked. "Why is this suddenly taking over? Why now?"

The timing is meaningful. If you've ever wondered why celery juice is making its way around the globe now and not at another moment in history, it's because we've never been as sick as we are in this modern age. It's at this moment in time that health is more challenged than ever by chronic symptoms and illnesses that hold people back in life. It's at this moment in time that people most need healing answers.

Would you ignore an offering that could change your life because of the source that offered it? We sometimes let our feelings dictate whether we choose to get help. "I'm not into that," we say. Or, "I don't believe that." If it really came down to an answer that could improve your life, would you let the calling override any initial unsure feelings about it? I've noticed people who stand in front of their 16 ounces of celery juice as nervous as if they're about to jump off a cliff into rough waters below. In their minds, they're battling their conditioning: the thought that celery is meaningless so drinking celery juice couldn't possibly hold any value. That thought alone can deter people from choosing to try it, which deters them from actually taking a step to heal. For some people, seeing celery juice reverse illnesses for others is not enough to get past their questioning of the source and their conditioning about celery's worth. Some people can only trust what comes out of a package and appears to be systematically tested and approved by some authority. Don't let that fear stop you from healing.

The truth about chronic illness has been so far away for so many decades, with good people researching and getting closer to answers. Famous neurologists get nearer to explaining what causes certain symptoms and conditions and then can't keep going due to lack of funding. Just as we get close in this modern day of medicine, in which so many people have suffered and even lost lives with no answers, all progress is put on the shelf. Answers are only *almost* found. A theory such as the gene blame game puts the truth further away, because it causes medical science to pour all its resources into researching genes instead of digging for the answers that would actually put a stop to the chronic illness madness that has been with us for far too long.

How many times have you seen something unfold that you knew could have gone differently if only others understood what you'd learned in life? For my whole life, I've watched the decades roll by while medical communities move along with steps and missteps, trying to figure out why people suffer. I've witnessed them almost stumble upon the answers to what causes chronic illness and then never quite pull through and succeed. My job is to deliver the answers to you, such as the healing power of celery juice. Are you ready to receive them?

I've been given the answers about chronic symptoms and conditions so that you don't need to be held back anymore by the blunders and roadblocks in the way of medical advancements in chronic illness. There are no funding deficits or agendas or grandfathered mistakes to stop you from discovering how to move forward, because I'm not shackled by a system. Freedom lives here in these words; it is attainable.

THE EPIDEMIC OF CHRONIC AND MYSTERY ILLNESS

Chronic illness is at an all-time high. In America alone, more than 250 million people are sick or dealing with mystery symptoms. These are people leading diminished lives with no explanation—or explanations that don't sit right or that make them feel even worse. You may be one of these people. If so, you can attest that medical science is still puzzling through what's behind the epidemic of mystery symptoms and suffering.

Let me be clear that I revere good medical science. There are incredibly gifted and talented doctors, surgeons, nurses, technicians, researchers, chemists, and more doing profound work in both conventional and alternative medicine. I've had the privilege of working with some of them. Thank God for these compassionate healers. Learning how to understand our world through rigorous, systematic inquiry is one of the highest pursuits imaginable.

Most doctors have an innate wisdom and intuition that tell them that the medical establishment doesn't give them what they need in order to offer the best diagnosis and treatment plan when it comes to chronic illness. How many times have you heard, "There is no known cure for [fill-in-the-blank disease]"? Even at the best, most elite medical schools, there are doctors who graduated at the top of the class who are honest about the fact that they finished school unprepared to work with chronic illness patients. They had to become experts on their own. Then there are doctors who believe that they are given all the answers in school and for some reason think that their training supersedes the mysteries of chronic illness; they think everything else is nonsense and hocus-pocus, which is unfortunate, since they live in denial of the millions of people who are suffering with no real answers. Either way, it's not doctors' or researchers' fault that the medical industry hasn't been able to solve the mysteries of chronic illness. Every day, amazing, brilliant minds in science stumble upon discoveries that require a green light from investors and decision makers at the top in order to move forward. Thousands of discoveries that could really change people's lives for the better are kept from going anywhere, and individuals in the field of science are held back.

We sometimes treat medical science like pure mathematics, governed solely by logic and reason. Though at times intertwined, math and medical science aren't the same. Math is definitive; science isn't. True science applies to an outcome, a result of applying theory. You can use math in medical science; you can use it to make a drug, for example, though the drug shouldn't be deemed scientific until there's a proven result and the numbers make sense in the end. Science labs are play shops of people methodically slapping together different materials to test out different hypotheses and theories while investors apply pressure to rush a favorable outcome. Too often, theories are treated as fact before they ever get a chance to be proven—or disproven. That's especially the case with chronic illness. It's extremely rare in the medicine of chronic illness that you ever get a straight answer that's correct.

Wouldn't it be nice if science were the ideal we sometimes make it out to be? If it were a pursuit where money never mattered and only the truth won out? Like any human pursuit, medical science is still a work in progress. Think about the recent recognition of the mesentery as an organ. Here this active, mesh-like connective tissue has been in plain sight all along and even acknowledged along the way, and only now is it beginning to get its full due. There's more to come; new breakthroughs occur every day. Science is constantly evolving, and so theories that one day seem like everything can be revealed the next day to be obsolete. Ideas that one day seem laughable can be proven the next to be lifesaving. What this translates to is: science doesn't have every answer yet.

We've already waited 100-plus years for real insights from medical communities into how people who live with chronic health problems can get better—and they haven't come. You shouldn't have to wait another 10, 20, 30, or more years for scientific research

to find the real answers. If you're stuck in bed, dragging through your days, or feeling lost about your health, you shouldn't have to go through one more day of it, let alone another decade. You shouldn't have to watch your children go through it, either—and yet millions do.

A HIGHER SOURCE

That's why Spirit of the Most High, God's expression of compassion, came into my life when I was four years old: to teach me how to see the true causes of people's suffering and to get that information out into the world. If you'd like to know more about my origins, you'll find my story in *Medical Medium: Secrets Behind Chronic and Mystery Illness and How to Finally Heal.* The short version is that Spirit constantly speaks into my ear with clarity and precision, as if a friend were standing beside me, filling me in on the symptoms of everyone around me. Plus, Spirit taught me from an early age to see physical scans of people, like supercharged MRI scans that reveal all blockages, illnesses, infections, trouble areas, and past problems.

We see you. We know what you're up against. And we don't want you to go through it a moment longer. My life's work is to deliver this information to you so that you can be elevated above the sea of confusion—the noise and rhetoric of today's health fads and trends—in order to regain your health and navigate life on your own terms.

The material in this book is authentic, the real deal, all for your benefit. This book is not like other health books. There was so much packed in here that you may want to come back and read it again to make sure you got all the information. Sometimes this information surely seemed to be the opposite of what you've heard before, and sometimes it sounded closer to other sources, with subtle and critical differences. The common thread is that it's the truth. It's not repackaged or recycled theory made to sound like a new understanding of chronic symptoms and illness. The information here doesn't come from broken science, interest groups, medical funding with strings attached, botched research, lobbyists, internal kickbacks, persuaded belief systems, private panels of influencers, health-field payoffs, or trendy traps.

The above hurdles get in the way of medical research and science making the leaps and bounds it's meant to in understanding chronic illness and what heals it. Think about this: If you're a scientist with a theory, once you've conjured that theory, you need to get investors. That means you need to pitch to them. If investors like your pitch, it's usually because they want to see a certain outcome, and so they fund your endeavor. This comes with incalculable pressure to produce favorable, tangible results and proof that justify the amount of money the investors poured into it. Scientists in this position are afraid that if they blow it, they'll never get another investor for another theory again, and their name won't hold any merit within the profession. That doesn't leave much space to follow what's supposed to be the natural path of inquiry: to have ideas not pan out sometimes, go in unexpected directions, or reveal that certain foundational beliefs are faulty. This constriction calls into question whether the reportedly breakthrough study results we read about are always quite as favorable as they report. When outside sources have a vested interest in obscuring certain truths, then precious research time and money get spent in unproductive areas. Certain discoveries that would truly advance the treatment of chronic illness get ignored and lose funding. The scientific data we think of as absolute can, instead, be skewed—contaminated and manipulated—and then treated by other health experts as law, even though it's inherently flawed. That's why trying to keep up with health information is so confusing and conflicting. Not all of it is truth.

Celery juice has already proven itself to be effective, tested in people's hands and people's homes with no agenda or funding to force a certain outcome. The documentation is only growing that celery juice is helping people. It's becoming more and more validated by the day. The millions of people getting better from celery juice, many of whom are changing nothing in their lives other than adding celery juice, take it out of the realm of the theoretical and into the domain of medical truth. In its original meaning, science is knowledge. I've seen no more certain knowledge than that in the eyes of someone who, after trying everything, has seen celery juice take them from bedridden to alive again.

To go with the facts and figures about celery juice and chronic illness that you just read throughout this book, you didn't find citations or mentions of scientific studies spawned from unproductive sources. You don't need to worry that this information will be proven wrong or superseded, as you do with other health books, because all of the health information I shared here comes from a pure, untampered-with, advanced, clean source—a higher source: the Spirit of Compassion. There's nothing more healing than compassion.

If you're someone who only believes in what science has to say, know that I like science, too. Also know that science still has a lot to learn. While we're in a great time, we're also sicker and more tired than ever before in history. If medical professionals had any idea what really causes people's suffering, there would be a revolution in the way we think about nearly every aspect of our health.

Unlike many other areas of science, which are strongly founded in weights and measures and math, scientific thinking about chronic illness is all still theoretical— and today's theories hold very little truth, which is why so many people are still dealing with chronic symptoms and conditions. If it keeps going like this, we'll reach a point where there won't be any studies at all in which agendas and interests aren't driving the outcomes against your favor. This trend is why the scientific establishment has let chronic illness communities down since the beginning, letting doctors down, too, and

leaving hundreds of millions to suffer. You don't need to be one of them.

WE THE QUESTIONERS

Once upon a time, we lived by the rule of authority. We were told that the earth was flat, and then that the sun revolved around the earth, so we believed it. Those theories weren't fact, and yet people treated them like they were. People living back then didn't feel like life was backward; it was just the way life was. Anyone who spoke out against the status quo seemed like a fool. Then came the paradigm shift of science. The questioners—the committed researchers and thinkers—the ones who all along hadn't been content to take a "fact" at face value, finally proved that analysis could open the door to a much deeper, truer understanding of our world.

Now, science has become the new authority. In some cases, this saves lives. Surgeons now use sterile tools, for example, because they understand the risk of contamination that surgeons of old didn't realize. Just because of certain advancements, though, we can't stop actively questioning. It's time for that next paradigm shift. "Because science" isn't enough of an answer when it comes to chronic illness. Is it good science? What was the funding behind it? Was the sample size diverse enough? Big enough? Were the controls handled ethically? Were enough factors considered? Were the measurement tools advanced enough? Does the analysis stamped on the results tell a different story from the numbers themselves? Was there bias? Did an influencer of establishment power put a thumb on the scale? Some science will hold up brilliantly. Some will reveal holes: payoffs, kickbacks, small sample sizes, poor controls. We're handed the word *science* as though we're meant to bow down to it without question. It sounds a lot like an authoritative ideology, doesn't it? We haven't shifted out of that belief system as much as we think. Progress doesn't happen without the very framework being questioned—and in our society today, we're not allowed to question the scientific framework.

Trends don't always look like trends. They often disguise themselves as sound medical advice. So much of the health information out there is repetition or, worse, garbled whisper-down-the-lane. We must be wary of someone sending out a message with an agenda so that when it reaches us, it's twisted. Good primary sources used to be the gold standard. Now, in an enormous push for content, some research for health literature gets rushed, published based on one okay-enough-sounding source. We must look at the special interests of who's interpreting and posting. Even the research results themselves—can they be trusted?

Science is so often used as an attack mechanism. That label can be used to put a spin on everything possible. Take the food wars, for example. Vegan and plant-based folks are battling paleo and keto folks with science. Paleo and keto folks are battling vegan and plant-based folks with science. They're both using studies to justify their sides—because you can find a study to justify practically anything. When even science isn't enough, food war participants go for the emotional aspect of the other's belief system. Vegan and plant-based folks tell paleo and keto folks they're killing animals. Paleo and keto folks tell vegan and plant-based folks they're starving themselves and their children. Regardless, they all encounter health challenges that neither they nor science understand. Getting better is not about choosing sides or what you have adopted as a belief system in that moment—even if it's a belief system based on reports you've read of scientific studies. It's about understanding our brains and bodies and supporting them in what they need.

We won't get there by treating science as God and treating those who question theories and findings as fools. Medical science looks out for medical science. While individual health-care providers can have the best of intentions, the greater industry is not about looking out for a person; it's about looking out for itself, since it has its authority to uphold. It's self-involvement in the most chronic way.

Let's be honest. Even today's science in those areas we think to be concrete sometimes shows cracks. If you've heard about recalls of hip replacement parts or hernia mesh, you know what I'm talking about. These are tangible items that were designed with exacting scientific standards, then went through rigorous scientific testing before being put to use, and even that highly scientific process wasn't guaranteed. Certain products developed unforeseen problems, and an area of science that seemed indisputable turned out to be fallible. Think, then, what kind of uncertainty remains in scientific understanding of chronic illness and how celery juice can alleviate it. Celery juice isn't a device that can be held in your hand, measured, and analyzed as solely independent from the rest of you. Once you drink it, it becomes an active part of the human body, and we all know the human body to be one of the greatest miracles and mysteries of life. If celery juice contains chemical compounds that science doesn't even know exist yet, and those compounds go after problems in our bodies that science doesn't know exist yet, how can we trust any source that says celery juice and its effects are lackluster? Again, science is a human pursuit and a work in progress, especially when that work involves decoding the human body. It takes constant vigilance, receptiveness, humility, and adaptability to keep that work truly progressing.

If you've never struggled with your health, suffering for years with no answers for your condition, or if you feel cemented within a certain medical, scientific, or nutritional belief system, I hope that you read these words with curiosity and an open heart. The meaning behind today's widespread chronic symptoms and suffering is so much bigger than anyone has yet discovered. What you've just read is unlike any information about chronic health issues or healing you've seen before. It's information that has helped millions of people over the past decades.

ALL IN THIS TOGETHER

Since I first started to share Spirit's information, I've been so blessed to see it make a difference for these people. With the publication of the Medical Medium book series, I've been beyond moved to see this information reach the wider world and help thousands more.

I've also noticed that some of these messages have been manipulated as certain career-driven individuals try to climb the ladder of acclaim and notoriety. This approach gets at people's core, raw nerve of suffering and takes advantage of it.

This is not how the gift I was given was ever meant to be used. Spirit is a voice for the ones in need of answers, a source independent from a system filled with traps that have wasted so many lives along the way. We love it when people become experts on the health information I share and when they spread the compassionate message far and wide in the name of truly helping others. I am so thankful for this. What gets dangerous is when that information is tampered with—intermixed and twisted with trendy misinformation, changed just enough so that it sounds original, or blatantly poached and attributed to seemingly credible sources that are anemic of the truth. I say this because I want you to know to protect yourself and your loved ones from the misguidance out there.

This book is not repetition of everything you've already read. It is not about a belief system that blames your genes or says your body is faulty, nor is it about putting a spin on a trendy high-protein diet to keep symptoms at bay. This information is fresh—an entirely new perspective on the symptoms holding back so many people in life, and an entirely new perspective on how to heal.

I get it if you're wary. We react, we judge; that's what we do. It can be an instinct that protects us in certain circumstances; sometimes, it gets us through life. In this case, I hope you'll reconsider. You may judge yourself out of learning the truth. You could lose the opportunity to help yourself or somebody else.

We are all in this together with getting people better, and I want you to become the new expert on celery juice. Thank you for coming with me on this healing journey and taking the time to read this book. Bringing the truths you've just read into your life will change everything for you and the ones around you—now you'll finally hold the knowledge and faith.

INDEX

Note: Page numbers in parentheses indicate intermittent references.

"If medical professionals had any idea what really causes people's suffering, there would be a revolution in the way we think about nearly every aspect of our health."

— Anthony William, Medical Medium

ACKNOWLEDGMENTS

Thank you to Patty Gift, Anne Barthel, Reid Tracy, Margarete Nielsen, Diane Hill, everyone at Hay House Radio, and the rest of the Hay House team for your faith and commitment to getting Spirit's wisdom out into the world so it can continue to change lives.

Helen Lasichanh and Pharrell Williams, you are extraordinarily kind-hearted seers.

Sylvester Stallone, Jennifer Flavin Stallone, and family, your support has been legendarily game-changing.

Jennifer Aniston, your kindness, caring, and support are on another level.

Miranda Kerr and Evan Spiegel, it's so amazing to have your hands of light and compassion behind the healing movement.

Novak and Jelena Djokovic, you are pioneers in advancing health and teaching the world how to thrive.

Gwyneth Paltrow, Elise Loehnen, and your devoted GOOP crew, your caring and generosity are a profound inspiration.

Dr. Christiane Northrup, your inexhaustible devotion to the health of womankind has become its own star in the universe.

Dr. Prudence Hall, your selfless work to enlighten patients who need answers renews the true, heroic meaning of the word *doctor*.

Craig Kallman, thank you for your support, advocacy, and friendship on this journey.

Chelsea Field and Scott, Wil, and Owen Bakula, how did I get so blessed to have you in my life? You are true crusaders for the Medical Medium cause.

Kimberly and James Van Der Beek, there's a special place in my heart for you and your family. I'm truly thankful to have crossed paths with you in this lifetime.

Kerri Walsh Jennings, you truly amaze me with your hopeful nature and endless positive energy.

John Donovan, it's an honor to be on the planet with such a peace-seeking soul.

Nanci Chambers and David James, Stephanie, and Wyatt Elliott, I can't thank you enough for your dear friendship and everlasting encouragement.

Lisa Gregorisch-Dempsey, your acts of kindness have been deeply meaningful.

Grace Hightower De Niro, Robert De Niro, and family, you are precious, gracious beings.

Liv Tyler, it's such a great honor to be a part of your world.

Jenna Dewan, your fighting spirit is an inspiration to behold.

Debra Messing, you are bettering people's lives with your vision for a healthy planet.

Alexis Bledel, your strength in this world is extraordinarily heartening.

Lisa Rinna, thank you for tirelessly using your influence to spread the message.

Taylor Schilling, what a joy to know you and have your support.

Marcela Valladolid, knowing you is a gift in my life.

Kelly Noonan and Alec Gores, thank you for always looking out for me. It means so much.

Erin Johnson, knowing you're there on my side is a blessing.

Jennifer Meyer, I'm beyond grateful for your friendship and how you're always spreading the word.

Calvin Harris, you've changed the world with a powerful rhythm.

Courteney Cox, thank you for having such a pure, loving heart.

Hunter Mahan and Kandi Harris, I'm proud of you for always being game to take on a challenge.

Peggy Lipton, Kidada Jones, and Rashida Jones, the deep care and compassion you bring to life mean more than you know.

Kris, Kourtney, Kim, Kanye, Khloé, Rob, Kendall, Kylie, and family, it's an honor to be part of the Kardashian-Jenner world that's helping so many.

To the following special souls whose loyalty I treasure, my thanks go out: Naomi Campbell; Eva Longoria; Carla Gugino; Mario Lopez; Renée Bargh; Tanika Ray; Maria Menounos; Michael Bernard Beckwith; Jay Shetty; Alex Kushneir; LeAnn Rimes Cibrian; Hana Hollinger; Sharon Levin; Nena, Robert, and Uma Thurman; Jenny Mollen; Jessica Seinfeld; Kelly Osbourne; Demi Moore; Kyle Richards; Caroline Fleming; India.Arie; Kristen Bower; Rozonda Thomas; Peggy Rometo; Debbie Gibson; Carol, Scott, and Christiana Ritchie; Jamie-Lynn Sigler; Amanda de Cadenet; Marianne Williamson; Gabrielle Bernstein; Sophia Bush; Maha Dakhil; Bhavani Lev and Bharat Mitra; Woody Fraser, Milena Monrroy, Midge Hussey, and everyone at Hallmark's Home & Family; Morgan Fairchild; Patti Stanger; Catherine, Sophia, and Laura Bach; Annabeth Gish; Robert Wisdom; Danielle LaPorte; Nick and Brenna Ortner; Jessica Ortner; Mike Dooley; Dhru Purohit; Kris Carr; Kate Northrup; Kristina Carrillo-Bucaram; Ann Louise Gittleman; Jan and Panache Desai; Ami Beach and Mark Shadle; Brian Wilson; Robert and Michelle Colt; John Holland; Martin, Jean, Elizabeth, and Jacqueline Shafiroff; Kim Lindsey; Jill Black Zalben; Alexandra Cohen; Christine Hill; Carol Donahue; Caroline Leavitt; Michael Sandler and Jessica Lee; Koya Webb; Jenny Hutt; Adam Cushman; Sonia Choquette; Colette Baron-Reid; Denise Linn; and Carmel Joy Baird. I deeply value you all.

To the compassionate doctors and other healers of the world who have changed the lives of so many: I have tremendous respect for you. Dr. Alejandro Junger, Dr. Habib Sadeghi, Dr. Carol Lee, Dr. Richard Sollazzo, Dr. Jeff Feinman, Dr. Deanna Minich, Dr. Ron Steriti, Dr. Nicole Galante, Dr. Diana Lopusny, Dr. Dick and Noel Shepard, Dr. Aleksandra Phillips, Dr. Chris Maloney, Drs. Tosca and Gregory Haag, Dr. Dave Klein, Dr. Deborah Kern, Dr. Darren and Suzanne Boles, Dr. Deirdre Williams and the late Dr. John McMahon, and Dr. Robin Karlin—it's an honor to call you friends. Thank you for your endless dedication to the field of healing.

Thanks to David Schmerler, Kimberly S. Grimsley, and Susan G. Etheridge for being there for me.

A very warm, heartfelt thanks to Muneeza Ahmed; Lauren Henry; Tara Tom; Bella; Gretchen Manzer; Kimberly Spair; Megan Elizabeth McDonnell; Ellen Fisher; Hannah McNeely; Victoria and Michael Arnstein; Nina Leatherer; Michelle Sutton; Haily Cataldo; Kerry; Amy Bacheller; Michael McMenamin; Alexandra Laws; Ester Horn; Linda and Robert Coykendall; Tanya Akim; Heather Coleman; Glenn Klausner; Carolyn DeVito; Michael Monteleone; Bobbi and Leslie Hall; Katherine Belzowski; Matt and Vanessa Houston; David, Holly, and Ginnie Whitney; Olivia Amitrano and Nick Vazquez; Melody Lee Pence; Terra Appelman; Eileen Crispell; Bianca Carrillo-Bucaram; Jennifer Rose Rossano; Kristin Cassidy; Catherine Lawton; Taylor Call; Alana DiNardo; Min Lee; and Eden Epstein Hill.

Thank you to the countless people, including those in the Medical Medium communities, whom I've had the privilege and honor of seeing blossom, heal, and transform.

Thank you to the Practitioner Support Group. Bless you for sharing the value of your experiences and carrying your teachings to others. You are changing the world.

Sally Arnold, thank you for shining your light so brightly and lending your voice to the movement.

Ruby Scattergood, your masterful patience and countless hours of dedication have heroically formed the true spine of this book. The Medical Medium series would not be possible without your writing and editing. Thank you for your literary counsel.

Vibodha and Tila Clark, your creative genius has been astoundingly instrumental to the cause of helping others. Thank you for standing with us throughout the years.

Friar and Clare: *Blessed is he that readeth, and they that hear the words of this prophecy, and keep those things which are written therein: for the time is at hand* (Rev. 1:3).

Sepideh Kashanian and Ben, thank you for your warm, loving care.

Ashleigh, Britton, and McClain Foster and Sterling Phillips, thank you for all your hard work and devotion. We're blessed to have you by our side.

Jeff Skeirik, thank you for the best pictures, man.

Jon Morelli and Noah, you two are all heart.

Robby Barbaro and Setareh Khatibi, your unwavering positivity lifts up everyone around you.

For your love and support, as always, I thank my family: my luminous wife; Dad and Mom; my brothers, nieces, nephews, aunts, and uncles; my champions Indigo, Ruby, and Great Blue; Hope; Marjorie and Robert; Laura; Rhia and Byron; Alayne Serle and Scott, Perri, Lissy, and Ari Cohn; David Somoroff; Joel, Liz, Kody, Jesse, Lauren, Joseph, and Thomas; Brian, Joyce, and Josh; Jarod; Brent; Kelly and Evy; Danielle, Johnny, and Declan; and all my loved ones who are on the other side.

Finally, thank you, Spirit of the Most High, for providing all of us with compassionate wisdom from the heavens that inspires us to keep our heads up and carry the sacred gifts you've been so kind to give us. Thank you for putting up with me over the years and reminding me to keep a light heart with your never-ending patience and willingness to answer my questions in search of the truth.

"People who have struggled with their health tend to hold pure hearts full of good intentions. They know what it's like to suffer. Celery juice is the perfect match for their honesty and purity of heart. It's elevated. Celery juice is a gift from the heavens, from God."

— Anthony William, Medical Medium

ABOUT THE AUTHOR

ANTHONY WILLIAM, the originator of the global celery juice movement and #1 *New York Times* best-selling author of *Medical Medium Liver Rescue: Answers to Eczema, Psoriasis, Diabetes, Strep, Acne, Gout, Bloating, Gallstones, Adrenal Stress, Fatigue, Fatty Liver, Weight Issues, SIBO & Autoimmune Disease*; *Medical Medium Thyroid Healing: The Truth behind Hashimoto's, Graves', Insomnia, Hypothyroidism, Thyroid Nodules & Epstein-Barr*; *Medical Medium Life-Changing Foods: Save Yourself and the Ones You Love with the Hidden Healing Powers of Fruits & Vegetables*; and *Medical Medium: Secrets Behind Chronic and Mystery Illness and How to Finally Heal*, was born with the unique ability to converse with the Spirit of Compassion, who provides him with extraordinarily accurate health information that's far ahead of its time. Since age four, Anthony has been using his gift to "read" people's conditions and tell them how to recover their health. His unprecedented accuracy and success rate as the Medical Medium have earned him the trust and love of millions worldwide, among them movie stars, rock stars, billionaires, professional athletes, and countless other people from all walks of life who couldn't find a way to heal until he provided them with insights from above. Anthony has also become an invaluable resource to doctors who need help solving their most difficult cases.

Learn more at www.medicalmedium.com

CONVERSION CHARTS

The recipes in this book use the standard United States method for measuring liquid and dry or solid ingredients (teaspoons, tablespoons, and cups). The following charts are provided to help cooks outside the U.S. successfully use these recipes. All equivalents are approximate.

Standard Cup	Fine Powder (e.g., flour)	Grain (e.g., rice)	Granular (e.g., sugar)	Liquid Solids (e.g., butter)	Liquid (e.g., milk)
1	140 g	150 g	190 g	200 g	240 ml
¾	105 g	113 g	143 g	150 g	180 ml
⅔	93 g	100 g	125 g	133 g	160 ml
½	70 g	75 g	95 g	100 g	120 ml
⅓	47 g	50 g	63 g	67 g	80 ml
¼	35 g	38 g	48 g	50 g	60 ml
⅛	18 g	19 g	24 g	25 g	30 ml

Useful Equivalents for Liquid Ingredients by Volume					
¼ tsp				1 ml	
½ tsp				2 ml	
1 tsp				5 ml	
3 tsp	1 tbsp		½ fl oz	15 ml	
	2 tbsp	⅛ cup	1 fl oz	30 ml	
	4 tbsp	¼ cup	2 fl oz	60 ml	
	5⅓ tbsp	⅓ cup	3 fl oz	80 ml	
	8 tbsp	½ cup	4 fl oz	120 ml	
	10⅔ tbsp	⅔ cup	5 fl oz	160 ml	
	12 tbsp	¾ cup	6 fl oz	180 ml	
	16 tbsp	1 cup	8 fl oz	240 ml	
	1 pt	2 cups	16 fl oz	480 ml	
	1 qt	4 cups	32 fl oz	960 ml	
			33 fl oz	1000 ml	1 l

Useful Equivalents for Dry Ingredients by Weight

(To convert ounces to grams, multiply the number of ounces by 30.)

1 oz	1/16 lb	30 g
4 oz	1/4 lb	120 g
8 oz	1/2 lb	240 g
12 oz	3/4 lb	360 g
16 oz	1 lb	480 g

Useful Equivalents for Cooking/Oven Temperatures

Process	Fahrenheit	Celsius	Gas Mark
Freeze Water	32° F	0° C	
Room Temperature	68° F	20° C	
Boil Water	212° F	100° C	
Bake	325° F	160° C	3
	350° F	180° C	4
	375° F	190° C	5
	400° F	200° C	6
	425° F	220° C	7
	450° F	230° C	8
Broil			Grill

Useful Equivalents for Length

(To convert inches to centimeters, multiply the number of inches by 2.5.)

1 in			2.5 cm	
6 in	1/2 ft		15 cm	
12 in	1 ft		30 cm	
36 in	3 ft	1 yd	90 cm	
40 in			100 cm	1 m

Hay House Titles of Related Interest

YOU CAN HEAL YOUR LIFE, the movie, starring Louise Hay & Friends
(available as a 1-DVD program, an expanded 2-DVD set, and an online streaming video)
Learn more at www.hayhouse.com/louise-movie

THE SHIFT, the movie,
starring Dr. Wayne W. Dyer
(available as a 1-DVD program, an expanded 2-DVD set, and an online streaming video)
Learn more at www.hayhouse.com/the-shift-movie

✱ ✱ ✱ ✱

MEDICAL MEDIUM: Secrets Behind Chronic and Mystery Illness and How to Finally Heal,
by Anthony William

*MEDICAL MEDIUM LIFE-CHANGING FOODS: Save Yourself and the Ones You Love
with the Hidden Healing Powers of Fruits & Vegetables,* by Anthony William

*MEDICAL MEDIUM THYROID HEALING: The Truth behind Hashimoto's, Graves',
Insomnia, Hypothyroidism, Thyroid Nodules & Epstein-Barr,* by Anthony William

*MEDICAL MEDIUM LIVER RESCUE: Answers to Eczema, Psoriasis, Diabetes, Strep,
Acne, Gout, Bloating, Gallstones, Adrenal Stress, Fatigue, Fatty Liver, Weight Issues,
SIBO & Autoimmune Disease,* by Anthony William

All of the above are available at your local bookstore,
or may be ordered by contacting Hay House (see next page).

✱ ✱ ✱

We hope you enjoyed this Hay House book. If you'd like to receive our online catalog featuring additional information on Hay House books and products, or if you'd like to find out more about the Hay Foundation, please contact:

Hay House, Inc., P.O. Box 5100, Carlsbad, CA 92018-5100
(760) 431-7695 or (800) 654-5126
(760) 431-6948 (fax) or (800) 650-5115 (fax)
www.hayhouse.com® • www.hayfoundation.org

———

Published in Australia by:
Hay House Australia Pty. Ltd., 18/36 Ralph St., Alexandria NSW 2015
Phone: 612-9669-4299 • *Fax:* 612-9669-4144 • www.hayhouse.com.au

Published in the United Kingdom by:
Hay House UK, Ltd., Astley House, 33 Notting Hill Gate, London W11 3JQ
Phone: 44-20-3675-2450 • *Fax:* 44-20-3675-2451 • www.hayhouse.co.uk

Published in India by: Hay House Publishers India,
Muskaan Complex, Plot No. 3, B-2, Vasant Kunj, New Delhi 110 070
Phone: 91-11-4176-1620 • *Fax:* 91-11-4176-1630 • www.hayhouse.co.in

———

Access New Knowledge.
Anytime. Anywhere.

Learn and evolve at your own pace
with the world's leading experts.

www.hayhouseU.com

Free e-newsletters
from Hay House, the Ultimate
Resource for Inspiration

Be the first to know about Hay House's free downloads, special offers, giveaways, contests, and more!

Get exclusive excerpts from our latest releases and videos from *Hay House Present Moments*.

Our *Digital Products Newsletter* is the perfect way to stay up-to-date on our latest discounted eBooks, featured mobile apps, and Live Online and On Demand events.

Learn with real benefits! *HayHouseU.com* is your source for the most innovative online courses from the world's leading personal growth experts. Be the first to know about new online courses and to receive exclusive discounts.

Enjoy uplifting personal stories, how-to articles, and healing advice, along with videos and empowering quotes, within *Heal Your Life*.

Sign Up Now!

Get inspired, educate yourself, get a complimentary gift, and share the wisdom!

Visit www.hayhouse.com/newsletters to sign up today!

HAY HOUSE

HAYHOUSE RADIO
radio for your soul®

HAYHOUSE
online learning

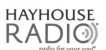

HAY HOUSE
Online Video Courses

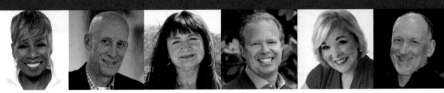

Your journey to a better life starts with figuring out which path is best for you. Hay House Online Courses provide guidance in mental and physical health, personal finance, telling your unique story, and so much more!

LEARN HOW TO:

- choose your words and actions wisely so you can tap into life's magic

- clear the energy in yourself and your environments for improved clarity, peace, and joy

- forgive, visualize, and trust in order to create a life of authenticity and abundance

- break free from the grip of narcissists and other energy vampires in your life

- sculpt your platform and your message so you get noticed by a publisher

- use the creative power of the quantum realm to create health and well-being

To find the guide for your journey, visit www.HayHouseU.com.

HAYHOUSE
online learning

"Once upon a time, we lived by the rule of authority. We were told that the earth was flat and then that the sun revolved around the earth, so we believed it. Anyone who spoke out against the status quo seemed like a fool."

— Anthony William, Medical Medium